Dr. Koeben
Thank you
all you do to
help children !

Stefanie
+
Remy

You Are What You
DON'T Eat

You Are What You DON'T Eat

How elimination diets saved my son's life, allowed me to reclaim mine and empowered my daughter to change the course of hers

---

Take Back Your Body LLC
Stefanie Sandler Billette, M.S., ACE-CHC

ISBN 978-1-73-513870-1

Take Back Your Body

I dedicate this book to my beautiful children- Rebecca and Remington. Being your mom is the greatest joy in my life.

CONTENTS

THE STORIES

STORY 1

HIS

Chapters:

STORY 2

MINE

Chapters:

STORY 3

HERS

STORY 4

YOURS

A.I.M.

You Are What You DON'T Eat

INTRODUCTION

Inherited metabolic disorders affect up to 1 in 1,000 newborns. According to the National Institutes of Health, up to 23.5 million Americans (nearly eight percent of the population) suffer from an autoimmune disease, and the prevalence is rising.

You Are What You DON'T Eat will guide readers like you who are desperate to improve the quality of life that has been stolen by the symptoms of chronic illness.

You Are What You DON'T Eat will take you on a journey of medical jigsaw puzzles that ends with your own story. This book is a conversation between you and me. It is a salvation that will help you manage (or even discover) your chronic illness, thus improving your individual quality of life and simultaneously reducing our collective burden on a medical system that is too reactive and has ignored the preventative power of diet on one's health.

By purchasing this book, you have decided to put your health first. You have made a choice to heal. I promise that you will not regret it.

STORY 1

HIS

Chapter 1

The NICU[1]

The NICU saved my son's life.

But, it also nearly killed him.

Remy was born seven weeks premature, weighing only 2 lb. 11 oz. He was delivered via C-section because he had stopped growing at twenty-seven weeks.

He came out with his arms up, in a boxer's stance. It was as if he knew he would be in for the fight of his life...a fight even harder than the one he had in the womb.

"He looks great. His Apgar is 9 and 9!" cheered the staff pediatrician, Dr. W.

I breathed a sigh of relief as my obstetrician began to sew me up. I thought to myself, "Wow, those shots of betamethasone[2] must have really worked these past two days!

[1] The NICU is the Neonatal Intensive Care Unit for premature or ill newborns.
[2] Betamethasone is a steroid given to mothers to speed up lung development in preterm fetuses who are at risk of being born too early.

"He weighs 2 pounds, 11 ounces", Dr. W continued.

Wow, I had thought Rebecca was tiny, weighing in at only 6 pounds, 6 ounces! Dr. W briefly brought Remy to my face so I could kiss him on the cheek. I could not move my body, so that would be the only contact I would have with him for a while.

C-sections are very bizarre. I don't know why anyone would *choose* to have one. You have just enough feeling to know you are being cut open but not enough feeling to actually move. I certainly hoped I would not need to have one, but I ended up having *two*. My amniotic fluid was so low with both my children that we had no choice. Remy was severely growth restricted in the womb and had to be delivered out at 33 weeks.

As soon as I was "put back together", I was taken to a room where I started pumping breast milk. It was several hours before I was wheeled into the NICU to see my precious little boy. There was my tiny son, in a plastic box with an IV in his head and an NG tube[3] in his nose.

All my life, I had been in such control of everything. I liked being in charge. I liked running the show. The moment I saw Remy – so tiny, so vulnerable - I instantly realized how little control I had over everything. This tiny human being, with whom I had already fallen in love, was at the mercy of both his fate and his physicians instead of being cradled in my arms as I had hoped and planned.

I knew that the only thing I could give him that no one else could was my colostrum. I knew that this would give him the best chance of growing strong so that he could come home with us. Giving him colostrum would give me a purpose while I alternated between sitting and pacing in my spacious, but empty, maternity suite.

He was immediately put on TPN[4], but I wanted to start giving him my colostrum as soon as possible. "Let the pumping begin", I thought as they wheeled me back to my room.

---

[3] Naso-gastric tubes are used to send food through the nose directly into the digestive system.
[4] Total Parenteral Nutrition is commonly given to preterm infants immediately after birth until full enteral feeds are established.

I am a very pragmatic person, so I was able to push aside any disappointment, sadness and fear at that moment because I had a job to do – pump, pump, pump. But, as I pumped, I also worried about my daughter who was almost seven-years-old. She was the center of our world as an only child for so long, and in an instant, all my attention had to be given to someone no bigger than a banana.

Remy was a bit of a surprise. I had trouble holding on to pregnancies. We had all but given up on having another child, but we weren't exactly doing a good job of preventing it. When we found out I was expecting again, we were filled with mixed emotions. We were much older than we were when we had Rebecca and not in a great financial situation, living on two teachers' salaries. We had spent all our savings so that I could stay home with Rebecca for her first two years and we never caught up.

When we had our ultrasound to see the sex of the baby, Rebecca asked if there was any possibility that the sonographer was pointing to an oversized nose instead of the clear indicator of his sex. She really wanted a sister.

The beginning of my pregnancy was uneventful, although I did have to go in for monthly appointments with a Maternal-Fetal Specialist since I was high-risk. I had frequent ultrasounds, and once they saw Remy's growth slowing at 27 weeks, I went in weekly. At 33 weeks, I was told he had to come out or he would not make it. They gave me steroid shots, and we scheduled a C-section. I had asked my OB if I should switch practices since hers only had privileges at our small local hospital, which had a Level 1 NICU[5], but she reassured me that everything would be fine and that she had delivered small babies before.

---

[5] All hospitals have at least a Level 1 NICU, which offers basic newborn care. Level II offers more advanced newborn care. Level III offers a full range of pediatric subspecialties for critical care. Level IV offers the highest level of acute neonatal care.

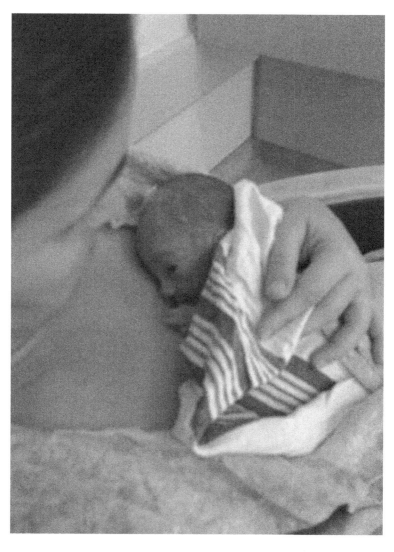

Remy, shortly after birth

Remy at 2 weeks old

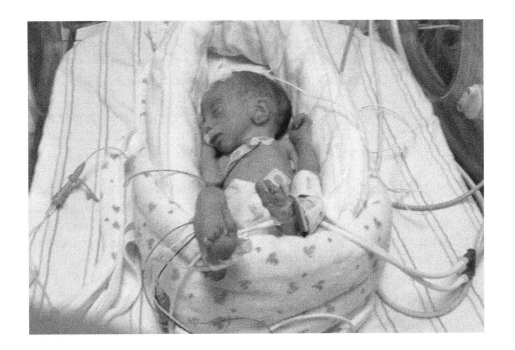

After Remy was born, I had to trust that my husband and my mother were giving Rebecca the care she needed while I was at the hospital. In the NICU, I pumped eight times a day and was given one hour per day to hold Remy. Skin-to-skin contact is so crucial to a NICU baby's development, especially when they spend twenty-three hours a day in a box. One hour of cuddles per day didn't feel like nearly enough time to hold my sweet baby, but my longing was quickly replaced by fear.

"His crit[6] is very low", said Dr. W, "he needs a blood transfusion."

I was shocked. How could he be anemic??? He was only a few days old! It didn't matter why, though, because his color was pale and his bradys[7] were frequent. We were not in a Children's Hospital, and I was starting to think we should transfer him. We decided to get the blood transfusion and then move him to a Level 3 NICU. I asked for a tour of the hospital's blood bank and was comforted, but I was still concerned since this was only the second blood transfusion they had ever done in this Level 1 NICU!

I began to do my usual online research. Time was of the essence, so we gave the go ahead for the transfusion. It took longer than it was supposed to, but he came through it without any obvious problems. I casually asked for confirmation that the blood had been irradiated[8] because I had read about this on the NIH website while the transfusion was taking place.

"No, we did not think it was necessary", Dr. W told me nonchalantly.

I was confused and terrified. I had read that very low birth-weight babies (i.e. under 1500 kg) should be given irradiated blood, and Remy was only

---

[6] "Crit" is short for hematocrit, which is the proportion, by volume, of the blood that consists of red blood cells. Low hematocrit indicates anemia.

[7] Part of the NICU vernacular, "bradys" are Bradychardias, slowed heart rates that indicate distress.

[8] Irradiated blood has been treated with radiation to prevent Graft-versus-Host Disease which is caused by white blood cells called lymphocytes in the transfused blood recognizing the patient as "foreign", leading to severe illness or even death.

1200 kg. The risk of graft-versus-host disease in premature infants is a rare complication of blood transfusions in which the immune system of the recipient identifies the donor blood as foreign; the body's strong defensive reaction can result in death.

I started to sob as I read that it can take thirty days for symptoms to begin. I imagined the next thirty days...watching my little love in an incubator as he struggles to grow, all the while fearing that he could die from the transfusion that was supposed to save him.

The doctor's reassurances did not help. The more questions I asked, the more I got the idea that they did not irradiate the blood because they had never transfused a newborn so tiny. A few hours after his transfusion, I told my husband, Shane, that we needed to transfer Remy to a Level 3 NICU immediately.

We moved in the middle of the night via a NICU transport ambulance. I had no appetite but knew I had to eat if I was going to continue to produce milk for Remy. When we arrived at the Level 3 Children's Hospital (which was 45 minutes from home), I realized that we were now small fish in a very big pond. We waited in a room with many other incubators until we were finally told there was a spot on the main floor.

Remy's incubator was wheeled into a tiny cubicle that was separated from the other incubators by a curtain. There were various alarms going off constantly, and it was impossible to relax. Being very germ-conscious, I organized my breast pump components on the small counter space only after I wiped it down thoroughly. I washed Remy's pacifier, which had been rolling around in his plastic space on the ride to the hospital (babies in the NICU get pacifiers immediately after birth to offer comfort since they get such little human contact).

We had no family living nearby, but my mom had driven four hours to stay with our daughter at home while my husband and I spent the first week in the NICU, 24-7. Now that we were at the Children's Hospital, we were not able to sleep there overnight, but we were told we could call anytime during the night to get updates.

"I want to stay here with Remy", I said as I wiped away a waterfall of tears.

"I know", Shane said with sympathy. "But, you need to come home to eat, shower, and sleep. You can come back first thing in the morning. We brought him here so you could trust that he would be in good hands, right?"

I left enough breast milk to get Remy through the evening. I would have to continue pumping every two hours throughout the night and come back first thing in the morning to make sure he had enough tomorrow.

It was 1 a.m. by the time we got home. One would think I could have drifted off immediately from sheer exhaustion, but instead my mind overpowered my body...

"What if he develops Graft vs. Host?"

"What if he needs another transfusion?"

"How is Rebecca going to handle having me away every day?

I finally fell asleep, but the alarm on my cell phone went off at 4 a.m.

Time to pump.

Shane got up with me and helped me wash the pump parts as I labeled and stored my milk in the refrigerator.

We went back to bed, and at 6 a.m., the alarm woke us up again.

"Pumping time", I muttered in a semi-conscious state as I stumbled down the stairs and into the kitchen. It was so strange to get up to an alarm and a plastic breast-pump instead of my sweet baby boy crying for me.

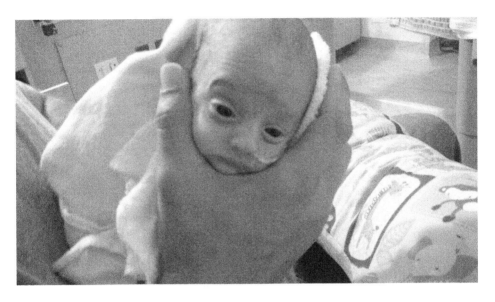

Remy, getting burped by Daddy in the NICU

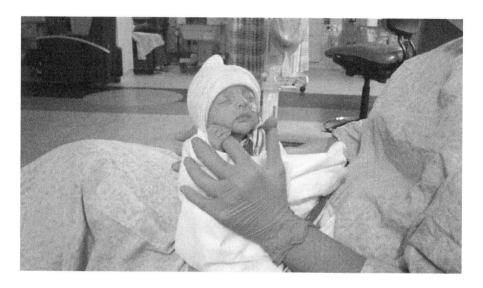

Remy, receiving therapy from an Occupational Therapist[9] in the NICU

[9] Occupational Therapists in the NICU help reduce the stressful conditions that the premature or ill newborn is exposed to as a result of psychological and physical immaturity. They help the newborn develop fine motor skills such as grasping an object.

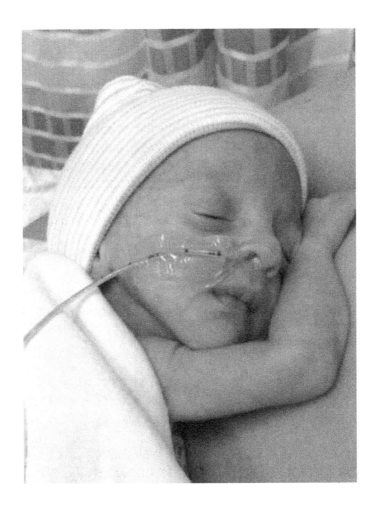

Remy & Me - Enjoying our one-hour of skin-to-skin contact per day

It was time to get Rebecca up for school and Shane out the door for work. My mom was going to pick her up from school so I could go to the NICU and spend the day there. I would come home in the late afternoon, spend a couple of hours with Rebecca, eat dinner, and then Shane and I would head back to the NICU together for a few hours in the evening while my mom stayed with Rebecca.

After a week of evaluations by every pediatric specialist, the consensus was that Remy would need another transfusion very soon. They said once a child is in the NICU, there are so many labs drawn every day that it is easy for their counts to drop. Since he had a transfusion shortly after birth, his body's production of red blood cells halted. His reticulocyte count [10] would be low for a while until his body recognized his increased demand.

The irony is that as soon as a transfusion is done, the reticulocyte rate drops because the bone marrow says, "OK, plenty of red blood cells now, so halt production", and so the cycle continues. In essence, blood was being taken from him faster than it was being made, so he was primed to become anemic again. Until the incessant blood draws stopped, I feared Remy would be on a never-ending loop to transfusions.

That week, Remy had his second blood transfusion at only three weeks of age. I felt relieved that at the Children's Hospital we were now in, irradiated blood was the standard for all NICU transfusions.

The problem was that Remy was still growing slowly and he had begun regurgitating frequently. His labs were starting to reveal several abnormalities with his liver function and bone health.

---

[10] Reticulocyte count measures how fast red blood cells are made by the bone marrow and released into the blood. It rises when there is a lot of blood loss or certain diseases in which red blood cells are destroyed prematurely, such as hemolytic anemia.

He had high bilirubin[11], low albumin, very high alkaline phosphatase[12], high transaminases, low Vitamin D and many more "out of range" values.

One day, when my husband and I were home for our brief time in the evening, we began to cry and prayed that God would let us bring our baby boy home.

"Please don't let him die in the hospital", Shane pleaded.

We were exhausted and scared. But, the NICU has a way of giving you the gift of gratitude. The next day, I was humbled as I watched other babies in the NICU struggle to breathe, undergo multiple surgeries, and eat through G-tubes[13].

There was a little girl next to Remy who never had any visitors. I was there sixteen hours a day and had never seen one person by her side. She looked very ill, and it broke my heart to see her all alone. One night, Remy's nurse, Courtney, told me her story.

"She was left here by her parents right after she was born. She has no family. We will take care of her until she is healthy enough to be placed in foster care and eventually gets adopted...*if* she gets healthy enough."

There was another baby who died while we were on the floor. The nurses cried briefly but had to move on to care for the dozens of other babies in their charge who needed to be fed, changed, poked, prodded and loved on.

---

[11] Bilirubin is an orange-yellow substance made during the normal breakdown of red blood cells. Bilirubin passes through the liver and is eventually excreted out of the body. High bilirubin may indicate different types of liver problems.

[12] Alkaline Phosphatase is an enzyme in a person's blood that helps break down proteins.
[13] A gastric tube is inserted directly into the stomach to provide nutrition to people who cannot obtain nutrition by mouth, are unable to swallow safely, or need nutritional supplementation.

When Remy turned seven weeks old, he hit the coveted 4 lb. mark. This is when a NICU baby can fit in a car seat and go home, provided s/he is healthy enough to do so.

Despite "making weight", the endocrinologists, gastroenterologists and hematologists[14] were still concerned about his labs. I argued that his health would improve at home with his family. I convinced the staff pediatrician to release Remy with the promise that I would follow up with each specialist in the next week.

We put our baby boy in his infant car seat, which looked like it was going to swallow him, and for the first time, the four of us headed home together.

---

[14] Endocrinologists specialize in hormonal and metabolic disorders; gastroenterologists specialize in organs of the digestive and elimination systems, such as kidneys, intestines, and liver; hematologists specialize in disorders of the blood and bone marrow.

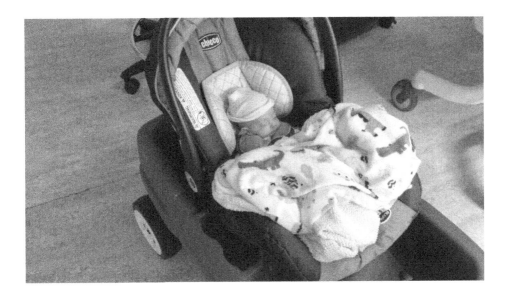

Remy at 4 lbs. and 7 weeks

Chapter 2
The Search

Over the next eighteen days, we tried to get into a routine. Shane went to work, Rebecca went to school, and I stayed home with Remy. My mom drove four hours south to her house, intending to come back up after a few weeks. I spent the days pumping milk, feeding Remy, and cleaning up the inevitable vomit that would come after each feeding.

Remy hardly slept, day or night, and I was surviving on adrenaline alone. Well, maybe not adrenaline alone. I started to drink one cup of coffee a day for the first time in my life just so I could make it through the day.

Remy did not look well. His skin and eyes were becoming the color of a lemon. Just three weeks after being released from the NICU, our concern became too great, so we took him back to the Children's Hospital, and he was admitted to the PICU[15] (once you are discharged from the NICU, there is no going back).

His liver enzymes were out of range. He was also anemic again and needed another transfusion. As expected, his hemoglobin and hematocrit rose after he was transfused, but his other labs remained worrisome. The doctors said they had never seen alkaline phosphatase in the 3000s before. They said his elevated bilirubin was abnormal and his stools were a worrisome color and consistency. His ammonia level was also elevated and this could lead to brain damage if untreated.

They wanted to rule out biliary atresia[16]. He would need to be given phenobarbital to prep for a HIDA Scan, which would allow them to view his

[15] The Pediatric Intensive Care Unit is for children up to age eighteen.
[16] Biliary atresia is a rare disease of the liver and bile ducts that occurs in infants.

liver. We were nervous about the test, but they reassured us that it was safe. The next morning, the nurse gave Remy his first dose of phenobarbital.

Within moments, I noticed Remy's eyes swelling.

"Nurse, something is wrong!"

The nurse examined Remy who was now looking like a marshmallow with puffy eyes, inflated hands and bloated feet.

The doctor rushed into Remy's room.

"I have never seen anyone allergic to phenobarbital. That is very rare", he said with surprise.

"So is our son, apparently", I replied impatiently.

Since Remy could not have any more phenobarbital, the HIDA scan would not be useful. A new gastroenterologist suggested we do "exploratory surgery". Shane and I scoffed at this suggestion.

"We will not put our son under anesthesia for a scavenger hunt", we replied as we left our local Children's Hospital and headed home.

We talked for hours with each other, our families, and our friends in the medical profession to figure out our next step.

After much research, my mother and I whisked Remy off to one of only two hepatologists[17] in Florida who was six hours away. Shane stayed home with Rebecca so they could continue some normalcy with work and school. I knew I would be missing both my daughter's 7th birthday and our 10th wedding anniversary, but there was no time to delay.

Dr. H was brilliant and compassionate; he encouraged me to continue pumping breast milk while other doctors had suggested we put Remy on

---

[17] A hepatologist is a sub-specialist in the specialty of gastroenterology who diagnoses and treats diseases of the liver and bile ducts.

formula. There is no doubt Remy would have died had I not followed my instincts and his advice. Remy's labs were not good; of particular concern to Dr. H was Remy's elevated PT/PPT.[18]

"Remy's PT/PTT levels are high which means he is at risk for a major internal bleed," Dr. H continued with his charming Cuban accent. "I believe all of these liver abnormalities are developmental due to his severe growth restriction in the womb. I am putting him on ursodiol, lactulose, vitamin K and Polyvisol. Vitamin K is a clotting factor that will help combat the elevated PT/PTT. Polyvisol will raise his hematocrit. Lactulose will bring down his ammonia and ursodiol with help his bile ducts."

This "cocktail" was designed to heal his sick liver.

Remy had blood drawn almost daily since his birth twelve weeks prior, so he needed a fourth blood transfusion while we were at the Children's Hospital under Dr. H's care.

After the transfusion, I noticed Remy was very calm...

"He is too calm", I though to myself. I moved closer to Remy and kissed his cheek. He was cold to the touch.

"Something is not right", I fearfully told my mom.

I called a nurse into the room.

"My son is not OK."

She glanced at Remy and immediately mirrored my alarmed face.

She checked his temperature.

---

[18] Prothrombin Time (PT) and Partial Thromboplastin Time (PTT) evaluate the overall ability to produce a clot in a reasonable amount of time.

95.8 degrees.

She checked his blood glucose.

36.

In the next two minutes, fifteen hospital staff members flooded the room and surrounded Remy. I broke down crying. One nurse put him under a heat lamp while another hooked him up to an IV. One doctor checked his vitals while two other people, who appeared to be administrators, were huddled and whispering with concern.

"Oh, God. My baby is going to die", I murmured with my hand over my mouth to stifle the wails that were battling to escape.

A nurse came up to me. "Remington is hypothermic and hypoglycemic. We are trying to get his temperature and blood sugar up before he goes into shock".

What followed was the longest twenty minutes of my life. I did not know if I would ever hold my baby boy again. I kept asking myself, "Did I kill him by bringing him here???"

After what felt like an eternity, a doctor spoke. "OK. His temp is up and glucose is stabilized".

I felt the blood flow back into my hands, feet and head. "How did this happen?" I asked myself, shaking.

Once everyone else had left the room, I approached the attending pediatrician.

"Why did he react this way to the blood transfusion?"

He said he would look into it.

An hour later, he came back and delivered another shocking blow.

"The blood was not warmed prior to his transfusion, so that could have contributed to his temperature dropping".

"How could you give him cold blood?"

"We did not think it was necessary to warm it."

This response was becoming all too familiar. My faith in hospitals was quickly waning, and once again, I felt a burning need to get him out of there and take him home where I could better protect him.

After three days in the PICU, Dr. H discharged Remy. We would continue to give him the "cocktail", and I would continue pumping breast-milk.

It had been an exhausting three months, but we were all hopeful that we were off the medical roller coaster and could start our life at home together.

Remy began to show signs of improvement over the next few months. We got him caught up on vaccinations, and despite his reflux, vomiting, diarrhea and inability to sleep for more than an hour at a time, we were grateful he was not in the hospital any longer. He vomited so frequently that my instincts were telling me to feed him every two hours to ensure he was getting enough nutrition.

When he was seven months old, I had to stop pumping because my supply disappeared. We put him on a hypoallergenic formula and he started to eat solids one at a time. On these new foods, he began to show signs of distress beyond the reflux and regurgitation. He still slept horribly, and I continued to get up with him multiple times. I would hold him all night most nights, and if I put him in the crib, I would sleep nearby to check on him. I would often find him in a cold sweat. I kept wondering if he was having a blood sugar issue. Sometimes, after he ate, it looked like he was waking from a coma. But, his lethargy would immediately turn to energy once he ate, and the cycle would continue.

He never seemed content. He was always hungry, then in pain, then he vomited. He would scream in the car, and I knew it was more than just reflux. So, we kept switching formulas. He did not take to solid foods easily. Rice cereal and oat cereal stayed down for the most part, but once we began introducing fruits and vegetables, he threw up even more than usual. Some foods he rejected outright (e.g. the mashed avocado shown on the cover of this book). He willingly ate bananas and prunes, but he immediately vomited them. I recorded every food and every reaction in the daily log that I had been keeping since the day he was born.

By eleven months old, his liver was quite enlarged and he looked like he had a potbelly. His jaundice was returning, and his ultrasound showed "lesions" that looked like "nothing we've ever seen" according to local radiologists and gastroenterologists. Again, doctors kept saying "liver biopsy" and "exploratory surgery". Aside from the inherent risks from surgery, he would need to fast for twelve hours prior to surgery.

"He cannot go even 4 hours without food", we insisted. There was no way we would let him go under the knife.

When Remy was a year old, we embarked on a journey that took us to multiple specialists. We saw nearly every gastroenterologist and geneticist in the state. Some would say, "let's do a liver biopsy", but most would order more labs, which brought along the fear of him becoming anemic again. All of the doctors had one thing in common- they each scratched their heads and said that nothing explained his unique array of symptoms.

One highly reputable doctor stands out as the most disappointing. I lugged my briefcase full of records into her office with Shane by my side, carrying Remy. When the doctor walked in, she looked at Remy, then at her nurse and said "Oh, that is an Alagille baby". At first, Shane and I felt a glimmer of hope when she uttered these words. But, I had read about Alagille Syndrome, and Remy did not seem to fit the profile.

He had many symptoms that were not explained by Alagille, so I had to speak.

"What makes you think he has Alagille?"

"Well, his dysmorphic facial features are a clear sign", she stated smugly.

It was true that Remy had the Alagille characteristics of a large head, low ears, large eyes and a small nose and chin. But, he also was severely growth restricted in the womb, vomited regularly and was still classified as malnourished, which was not explained by Alagille.

I hoped that she would dig a bit deeper. I spent two hours explaining and presenting Remy's medical history. She took copies of everything and said she would spend the weekend at home looking over all his labs, scans and notes and would call us after reviewing the piles of files.

We never heard from her again. When I called her office, I was told she no longer had the time for our case.

Chapter 3
The Answer

At my annual ob-gyn check-up, I told my physician (who was educated in the UK) what we had been through with Remy and what his symptoms were.

"Has anyone mentioned Glycogen Storage Disease?" Dr. S asked.

"No, what is that?" I was intrigued.

"GSD is a rare metabolic disorder caused by enzyme deficiencies that can damage liver cells, cause poor growth, and lead to feeding difficulties as well as hypoglycemic episodes" Dr. S. explained.

This sounded just like Remy!

I could not contain my excitement and gave Dr. S a huge hug as I left his office. I went home to my familiar NIH searches and began reading about GSD. I also read information about Hereditary Fructose Intolerance[19] (a.k.a. Fructosemia), which was similar to GSD but explained Remy's elevated bilirubin. He had other lab results and symptoms that were not explained by either disease, but these diseases seemed to present most similarly to his primary symptoms.

Both GSD and HFI are treated through dietary modification. For HFI, the diet is 100% fructose-free. This involves much more than just eliminating fruits. Fructose is found in all fruits, vegetables, legumes, nuts, seeds, whole grains, spices and sweeteners. Being fructose-free automatically means that one has to be sucrose-free because sucrose is a disaccharide, which consists

---

[19] Hereditary fructose intolerance (HFI) is a metabolic disease caused by the absence of the enzyme Aldolase B. In people with HFI, ingestion of fructose (fruit sugar), sucrose (which includes table sugar) or sorbitol (which is converted to fructose in the body) causes severe hypoglycemia (low blood sugar) and the build up of dangerous substances in the liver.

of fructose and glucose. So, all "sweets" such as table sugar, honey, and molasses are off-limits.

GSD Type 1 (the most common type) is treated by restricting fructose, sucrose and lactose in one's diet and by drinking cornstarch mixed with water throughout the day to maintain normal blood glucose levels.

With both disorders, sugars get trapped in the liver and symptoms include an enlarged liver (hepatomegaly) and hypoglycemia.

Since I did not know whether Remy had GSD or HFI, I decided to give him regular doses of cornstarch and strictly eliminated all the possible sources of sucrose, fructose, lactose and sorbitol.

Our little boy was eighteen months old, and we were tired of having no answers...

A diet that is 100% fructose, sucrose and lactose-free is difficult, to say the least. Sugars are everywhere. It took me a month of sorting through the wrong information from dietitians who knew nothing about HFI or GSD to finally get all the sugars out of his diet. We put him on a fructose-free / lactose-free amino acid formula that cost $1000/month, and I prepared all his foods from scratch to guarantee they were safe. I became more and more convinced that he had HFI, but I decided to keep him lactose-free as well just to be on the safe side.

The change in Remy was miraculous. He immediately stopped projectile vomiting. He went from having no teeth at thirteen months old to getting two or three teeth at a time. His stools became normal and his severe diaper rash became a thing of the past. His hair grew. He began sleeping for more than two hours at a time. His hypoglycemia nearly disappeared, and he was no longer yellow.

Clinical evidence confirmed what we were witnessing. Remy's belly shrunk and his blood work improved. His ultrasound showed that those mysterious liver "lesions" stopped growing for the first time.

But, he still ate like a bird and was nowhere near being on the growth charts.

We had already made two appointments prior to putting him on the diet. We wanted a definite answer. Without a diagnosis, how could we know the progression of his condition?

We went out of state to a clinic for rare diseases at one of the top children's hospitals in the nation. We met with a team of experts who said they had never seen anything like this. They all agreed something was not right, but they had no idea what it could be. They recommended genetic testing, and if nothing was found, they suggested a biopsy. They wanted to start with a few specific tests and would eventually get to more comprehensive (i.e. more expensive) tests. I wanted to test for HFI immediately, but they said that was not their first test. It would be months before we had results, and we would likely have to battle our insurance company to cover it, just as we had to fight for coverage of Remy's million dollar medical expenses over the past eighteen months.

When we returned home, we saw a medical geneticist with whom I had made an appointment three months earlier. He was known for being a brilliant diagnostician who could solve the most complex genetic puzzles. We hoped he would have some theories while we waited for genetics results.

Dr. P was friendly, funny, and confident (but not condescending like so many of the doctors we had met before). He poured over my briefcase full of Remy's medical records and the daily food logs I kept since day one. I gave him a summary of the journey we had been on the past year and a half.

"Are you in the medical field? Dr. P asked.

I responded as I always did when asked this question.

"No, but I was a pre-med drop-out, much to my mother's dismay."

Dr. P was one of a handful of American doctors who was considered an expert in HFI, so I felt strongly that we were finally in the right hands. I told him about the diet that we had started three months earlier. He was pleased that Remy's serious symptoms had abated, but he was concerned about his slow growth. In fact, Remy was still not on the charts and some of his development was slow. While he met many of his milestones, his verbal skills were lacking, he was still on bottles of formula for 80% of his nutrition, and he looked like he was half his age. Remy was getting all necessary nutrients from his amino acid formula, but Dr. P felt he needed more.

"I am putting him on Levocarnitine. This particular amino acid will heal the mitochondria and help him grow." Dr. P explained, "I want to see him back in three months to measure his growth and re-do his labs."

In the mean time, Dr. P ordered the test for HFI.

Six weeks later, the HFI test came back negative! This did not make any sense to me. Remy's symptoms had improved markedly on the HFI diet.

Within a six-month period, we had many more genetic tests come back from the rare diseases clinic. None of the genetic tests gave us a diagnosis. There were no other tests out there! This was the extent of what was currently available in the world of genetic sequencing.

The experts at the rare disease clinic concluded "There is no need for Remy to continue on a restricted diet since the metabolic tests were negative". My instincts told me otherwise, so I kept him fructose-free.

We were baffled by the lack of a diagnosis. It was clear that the switch to fructose- free was helping. He was taking the amino acid formula and holding it down. I even added some dairy into his diet and he seemed to do all right with the lactose.

I ensured that all his foods were "HFI safe", yet he would eat a few bites of whatever I offered and refuse to eat more. After eighteen months of vomiting, food was not his friend.

There was some improvement. He was sleeping five hours straight at night for the first time ever. He was not in constant pain. He started to talk more. We HAD to be on the right track. I was certain that Remy could not metabolize fructose. I recalled one time when he was only a year old, we gave him Ibuprofen for his first fever. Children's Ibuprofen contains sorbitol, and he got so sick after taking it that he looked like death. Sorbitol gets converted to fructose in the body and is seven times more toxic to the HFI liver than fructose. Surely, this experience was proof that he could not process fructose.

Genetic testing did reveal one thing. He was a carrier for GSD 1b. I asked the geneticists if he could be a GSD 1b carrier who shows serious symptoms due to a combination of factors. While they said this is impossible, I have considered the statistics.

Being severely IUGR due to pathology is rare.

Being Very Low Birth Weight (VLBW) is rare.

Having an allergic reaction to phenobarbital is rare.

Having an inborn error of carbohydrate metabolism is rare.

At this point, the word "rare" means very little to us. Remy has been "rare" so often that nothing seems improbable at all.

In search of answers, I joined the HFI message board, which is an excellent support group for those with HFI and their families. Like some others on the board, I relayed that my son has every symptom of HFI yet genetic testing for HFI came back negative. I called the lead researcher of HFI in the United States, and after hearing Remy's story, he concluded that our son has must have an HFI mutation that has yet to be identified.

One puzzle piece still didn't fit.

Most children don't get diagnosed with HFI until they start table foods or infant formula that contains sucrose. Yet, Remy's liver symptoms started in the NICU while he was on breast milk. From the day he was born, I kept a daily journal, which detailed when and how much he ate, whether he got sick afterward, and how he looked and acted. My lifetime of record-keeping was paying off as I started to see some patterns.

I had reiterated to doctors from the beginning that he gets hypoglycemic, to which they would reply, "That's because he's tiny". I always thought that he was more than "just tiny".

"How did he develop jaundice and other liver issues as a newborn on breast milk in the NICU?" I kept wondering.

That is when the light bulb went off. "Was he given something else besides my milk???"

Then, I remembered that the nurses gave him a syringe of liquid *every time* they drew his blood. It was the method they used to calm the babies. I called the NICU manager and found out that the "Sweet Ease" that is given to NICU babies is, in fact, pure sucrose. This realization sent my mind into a tailspin. The doses of sugar water explained his early fructose exposure and liver damage! I was even more convinced by this revelation that my little guy indeed had HFI.

The irony of this cycle hit me like a freight train. Our son had been given sugar to calm him for blood draws. As his labs worsened, more labs were drawn and the more sugar he was given! He had essentially been poisoned with the very thing that was causing him to be ill in the first place in an attempt to diagnose him!

I quickly launched a petition to stop the practice of giving NICU babies sucrose since thousands of babies have undiagnosed metabolic disorders and sucrose could pose great danger to them.[20] Manufacturers of infant formula have recently been pressured to remove sucrose from infant formula and the NIH is now connecting the dots between SIDS and underlying metabolic disorders. [21]

[20] https://www.change.org/p/american-hospital-association-get-sugar-water-out-of-the-nicu
[21] https://www.sciencedaily.com/releases/2018/05/180517142518.htm

I sent letters along with my petition to the manufacturer of the sugar water, the hospitals, and even news outlets. Not one of them has responded to date.

Dr. P has discovered 40+ genetic diseases in his decades of practice, and he explained that we can only test for what we know. He has no doubt that our son has something rare - so rare that it is possible no one else has ever had it or no one else has ever survived long enough to make it known.

Our little boy clearly has a form of HFI. Dr. P has officially diagnosed him with "a defect in carbohydrate metabolism at the mitochondrial level with carnitine deficiency".

Fructose was depleting Remy's cells of ATP (cellular energy), and putting Remy on carnitine (which helps stimulate ATP), finally allowed his body to absorb nutrients and grow. At age three, he was finally on the charts for weight and height!

While his metabolic symptoms disappeared and he began to eat more solid food, he also started to have more frequent croup-like coughs. He gagged and vomited because he produced excess phlegm. I began to wonder if he had a compromised immune system.

Antonia, one of the moms I had become friends with on the HFI message board who also happened to be a food scientist, told me her daughter not only had an HFI-like disorder (she, too, tested negative on genetic tests), but also had Eisonophilic Esophagitis (EOE)[22] triggered by wheat. Remy's eosinophil level had always been high, so Antonia suspected that a wheat allergy was a plausible explanation for his chronic respiratory symptoms.

---

[22] EOE is an immune response that is usually triggered by certain foods or environmental allergens and causes GERD-like symptoms.

I eliminated wheat from Remy's already limited diet when he was 4 ½ years old. Within a few days, I noticed a dramatic improvement. Days passed, weeks passed, months passed...no more croup, no more phlegm, no more cough, no more gagging!

Remy's medically restricted diet is working, as evidenced not just by his outward appearance but also with improved labs and ultrasound imaging. He has labs so frequently that we are able to see dips and changes in his complicated chemistries that indicate his body is trying to heal but has relapses at times. He only gets hypoglycemic with high fever, and I have been able to keep him hydrated even through some scary childhood illnesses (e.g. "Hand, Foot, and Mouth Disease"). After months in hospitals as an infant, my goal is to keep him out of one.

Remy no longer has a potbelly and he is accepting "safe" foods more each day. As he gets older, he will be able to tell us more and a lot of the guessing will go away. He eats the same ten foods all the time. I make him "goat kefir muffins" and "oat milk popsicles" as special treats, and he happily eats them while friends gobble down cupcakes at birthday parties. He never complains. On some level, his body seems to know and tells him "that will make you ill".

Remy's diet consists of meats, fish, dairy and a few carbs such as oats and white rice. I make him batches of oatmeal crackers with tapioca starch, cornstarch, white rice flour, oat flour, and butter. I prepare fructose-free, gluten-free pancakes, waffles, and bread and freeze huge batches for him. I order safe beef, bacon and poultry from grasslandmeats.com to fill up my deep freezer. I make him jerky using my food dehydrator and make him safe soups and stews from scratch.

Remy is starting to like food more. He understands that he cannot eat "fruits, vegetables or any form of sugar" as he says. He used to say "food makes my tummy hurt", but recently, I have seen him actually enjoy eating, and that makes me so happy. Those early experiences stick with us, and it took a long time for him to trust any food other than his bottles of amino acid formula.

He is a happy kid who knows what is good for his body. At five years old, he was able to start school for the first time. He sat at the food allergy table and I checked on him mid-day. He is a fantastic soccer player and will go up to anyone and start talking, singing and dancing.

He is not a deep sleeper. I believe the early days of NICU alarms and hypoglycemic episodes set the stage for poor sleep patterns. I was always a light sleeper and after those days in the NICU, awaking to an alarm every two hours and sleeping by his side, I thought I would never sleep well again. But, once he turned five, he started sleeping through the night.

Remy is rare. He is, in fact, the rarest of the rare. I have met so many fantastic people being part of a network of rare kids and their parents. I have forged friendships with people who live across the country and across the world, most of whom I will never meet. While our stories are all unique, we share a common link of fear, love, perseverance and hope. I wrote Remy's story for the Rare and Undiagnosed Network[23] a while ago and this was the impetus for my decision to write this book. I want people to know they are not alone and that there is an answer out there.

Having a treatment that is working in the absence of a firm diagnosis tells us we are on the right path toward keeping Remy healthy and helping his liver heal. But, we know that this is an unpredictable journey. It can be scary to not know exactly what his future holds. We live in a world where candy is thrown at children as a reward for answering math problems correctly. Fructose and sucrose are everywhere, including medications and vaccines.

I bring Remy's homemade foods and specially compounded supplements and medications wherever we go. He wears a medical ID necklace to communicate his condition in case of an emergency.

Food is not the center of his life. He eats to live, not the other way around.

---

[23] https://rareundiagnosed.org/rarest-rare-our-miracle-boy-stefanie-b/

We still don't know by what mechanism fructose makes him so ill. There are thousands of pathways in fructose metabolism and we have not identified where he has an error, but what we do know is that he is strong, brave, happy, smart and full of energy. We know he is loved beyond measure and that he has the people he needs around him to keep him healthy.

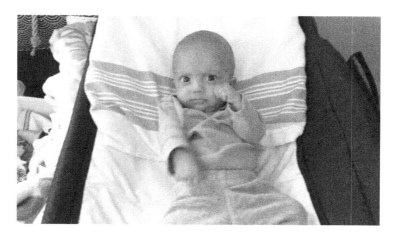

Instead of whining and feeling sorry for himself when he doesn't feel well, he just gets downright mad. He was a fighter from day one and still is.

STORY 2

MINE

Chapter 1
The Diagnosis

When I was eleven years old, I "blossomed" long before any of my friends...and I was excited when it happened (what was I thinking?!).

In hindsight, this was the year that set my destiny. In the springtime, I contracted mononucleosis. I shared food and drinks with friends regularly, so I am sure that is how I inadvertently got "the kissing disease".

In one year, I went from a lean, vibrant girl with thick dark hair and clear skin to a chubby, lethargic pre-teen with thinning follicles and cystic acne. I also developed tiny bumps ("KP" or keratosis pilaris[24]) all over my upper arms and thighs. My periods were horrible. I had chronic sinus infections. I started to have chronic headaches, bloating and my vision changed. One of my more bizarre symptoms was the tendency to get a splotchy red rash all over my chest and neck any time I had a viral infection. Quite predictably and repeatedly, I would get a sore throat, then a stuffy nose, then my itchy, burning rash which spread from my chest to behind the ears, and finally, a sinus infection, for which I would be given antibiotics. I had itchy ears, a painful scalp and a puffy white tongue. My lips would get red, burn and peel.

In the midst of all this, I decided I no longer wanted to eat meat at the age of thirteen. While all my future life-altering decisions would be based on serious research and contemplation, my teenage vegetarianism was based solely on a movie called *City Slickers* in which there was an adorable calf named Norman whom I decided I could never eat.

---

[24] Keratosis Pilaris is a skin condition that causes dry, rough patches and tiny bumps, usually on the upper arms, thighs, cheeks or buttocks.

I did not balance my meals well and my mom begged me to rethink my restricted diet at such a critical age, but I was stubborn and refused. I filled my plate with brown rice, beans and tofu. This would turn out to be a huge mistake.

My ophthalmologist detected visual disturbances and sent me for an MRI, which identified a microadenoma (small, non-cancerous tumor) on my pituitary gland. He referred me to an endocrinologist.

I will never forget walking into Dr. L's office to go over my labs, with my parents seated on either side of me.

"Well," Dr. L started without, making eye contact with any of us. "You have the labs of an 80 year-old".

Once my parents and I got over the shock of his statement, my mother begged, "What do you mean?"

"Her hormones are all out of whack. Her thyroid antibodies are sky high, her TSH is elevated, her vitamin levels are all off, and she has nodules on her thyroid that we need to check as well. I need more labs".

We left Dr. L's office confused, sad, and angry.

My parents, both psychologists, had divorced when I was three. I was an only child, a straight-A student, a tennis player, and a volunteer at the local hospital. They generally worked well together when it came to my health and my education. I gave them little to worry about...until now.

The news that their teenage daughter was having medical problems was shocking, but they agreed that I needed to get as many tests and labs done to figure out how to treat my condition. After many more labs, Dr. L diagnosed me with Hashimoto's Thyroiditis[25] and put me on Synthroid, synthetic thyroid hormone replacement. The thyroid is responsible for so

---

[25] Hashimoto's disease is an autoimmune disorder that can cause hypothyroidism, or underactive thyroid. With this disease, your immune system attacks your thyroid, preventing it from making enough thyroid hormone.

many functions such as metabolism, growth and development. Surely, taking thyroid hormone would make me feel better!

Despite taking Synthroid, few of my symptoms improved (in fact, most of them worsened) until a new doctor suggested putting me on birth control pills (even though I was not sexually active). She said it would help with my acne, PMS, and the length and severity of my periods. So, at age sixteen, I started what would be a decade-long dosing of birth control pills.

She was right about improving my acne and the regulating my periods, but I had no idea until much later how much of a toll those pills would take on me in other ways by increasing my risk of blood clots and causing vitamin deficiencies[26]. At age eighteen, I went away for college and continued to battle fatigue, bloating and many other symptoms that had begun years earlier.

[26] https://thyroidpharmacist.com/articles/14-ways-birth-control-pills-rob-us-of-our-health/

Chapter 2
The Struggle

After many years together, Shane and I got married when we were twenty-six, and soon we decided we wanted to have a family. I got off birth control pills, immediately and begrudgingly welcoming my familiar long, painful, irregular cycles and my unsightly blemishes.

I got pregnant very quickly. But, our excitement was dashed at nine weeks when we went in for an ultrasound and were told that the baby's heartbeat had stopped. The doctor came in to tell me even more distressing news.

"We detected another baby that had not been visible before and seemed to have died much earlier. You had identical twins", Dr. Y told us. "I am sorry; but they appear to have been conjoined. This is very rare and does not have a good outcome in most cases".

Shane and I went home and cried for hours.

The next day, I went in for a D&C[27] and with that, my twins were gone.

A few months later, I was pregnant again. This time, I was put on progesterone as soon as my pregnancy was confirmed. Everything looked good at my six-week ultrasound, but a few days later, I started to bleed. I knew that I had lost the baby.

We decided to take a break from "trying" and focus on other things. But, after a while, it was time to try again. At age twenty-eight, I got pregnant for the third time, and we were very cautious with our enthusiasm. Even as we saw this beautiful child growing and got more reassurance with each

---

[27] Dilation and curettage (D&C) is a procedure to remove tissue from inside the uterus.

ultrasound, we were scared that we would lose our baby girl.

Twice per week, I went in for my fetal monitoring. I was considered high-risk after two miscarriages and abnormal genetics results, which revealed two inherited risk factors (an MTHFR mutation and a Factor V Leiden mutation) that made me prone to pregnancy-related issues[28]. I was put on low-dose aspirin to help prevent clots in the placenta that are more probable with a Factor V Leiden mutation. I was also put on a very high dose of B12 and folate to keep my homocysteine level down (which can be elevated in those with MTFHR mutations and also lead to blood clots). I was also instructed to inject Lovenox, a blood thinner, into my growing uterus each day.

At thirty-nine weeks, my anxiety rose. "Your amniotic fluid is very low. We can try to induce you and if that does not work, we can do a C -section in two days, or we can just do a C-Section today and get her out".

After our losses, my husband and I chimed in unison, "Get her out today".

Our precious Rebecca was born healthy at 6 lb. 6 oz. with fair skin and big eyes. I was instantly in love. She looked just like my husband and had none of my olive skin, dark brown eyes and brown hair. I hoped that perhaps since she looked like Shane, she would be spared the health curses with which women on my side of the family were plagued.

Shane and I were both teachers, so the plan was for me to go back to teaching middle school math after a three-month maternity leave. Well, we all know what they say about the best-laid plans...

Breastfeeding did not go well, and after just six weeks, Rebecca had to go on formula. I was very depressed and couldn't shed the pregnancy weight, and once I finally went in for my check up, we discovered my TSH[29] was 12! I was VERY hypothyroid. No wonder I was sad, fat, had acne and was always

---

[28] https://www.ncbi.nlm.nih.gov/pmc/articles/PMC4877892/

[29] TSH stands for "thyroid stimulating hormone" and the test measures how much of this hormone is in your blood. TSH is produced by the pituitary gland in your brain. This gland tells your thyroid to make and release the thyroid hormones into your blood. High TSH indicates a sluggish thyroid. Low TSH reveals an overactive thyroid.

freezing. The endocrinologist raised my Synthroid dose significantly. Yet, I continued to have my usual array of symptoms...itchy ears, sore and swollen tongue, rashes, and inexplicable panic attacks. At the age of thirty, I was starting to feel like that eighty year-old woman Dr. L recognized many years ago.

I couldn't bear the thought of going back to work and leaving Rebecca. After seeing how happy I was in my profession, my husband had left the banking industry only a year earlier to become a teacher. If I stayed home with Rebecca, how were we going to live on only one teacher's salary?

I did not go back to my teaching position after maternity leave. Instead, I started teaching college courses online part-time and tutored three nights a week. Shane and I would often high-five when he walked in the door from work at 4 p.m. and I would immediately leave while he took care of Rebecca at night. It was hard, but not as hard as leaving her in daycare would have been.

After three months on my new Synthroid dose, I was having palpitations, sweating profusely, losing weight and feeling very anxious. My TSH was now 0.04. Clearly, my dose was too high and I was very hyperthyroid. We tried to find a happy medium between the two doses, but I never felt quite right and my TSH was never where I wanted it to be, falling between 2.5 and 3, which was considered normal but was definitely not ideal for me.

When Rebecca was twenty-two months old, she started daycare and I went back to teaching full-time. It was around this time that I read about non-celiac gluten sensitivity.

Bloating...check.
Stomach pain...check.
Constipation....check.
Brain fog...check.
Fatigue....check.
Numbness in fingers and toes....check.

There seemed to be a correlation between autoimmune diseases and gluten sensitivity that was being observed anecdotally.

While Hashimoto's Thyroiditis is one of the most common autoimmune diseases (especially among women), there are many other autoimmune diseases. When someone has an autoimmune disease, the immune system mistakes "self" as "foreign" and sends out autoantibodies to attack either a particular organ or the whole body (systemic). Healthy cells are destroyed in the process[30]

Doctors do not understand why this happens but they know that some people are more prone to autoimmune conditions than others, some autoimmune diseases tend to run in families, and women develop autoimmune diseases at twice the rate of men. Researchers believe western diets, environmental toxins, infections and genetics all play a role in who gets an autoimmune disease and at what age.[31]

I decided to give it a whirl and go gluten-free. Within six months, my bloating and gas improved dramatically. Many other symptoms improved as well. In fact, one symptom, Keratosis Pilaris, which was not even mentioned as being connected to gluten, nearly vanished!

Gluten was definitely out of my life forever. I lost some weight since I was eating less carbs in general. But, as gluten-free quickly became trendy, more gluten-free treats and cheats like desserts and pizzas became readily available. This was not a good thing. I substituted all kinds of gluten-free breads, cereals, and desserts and probably ate more of it than I should have. I was always vacillating between lean and a bit overweight. In particular, I always gained weight in my mid-section. I did not feel bloated anymore, but I still wanted to lose 10 lbs. I still had acne and many other unpleasant symptoms.

[30] www.healthline.com/autoimmunedisorders
[31] https://pathology.jhu.edu/autoimmune/classification

When Rebecca was four, we found out that I was pregnant again. We were not trying, per se. But, we were excited as we approached the end of the first trimester.

I was at a bridal shower for a friend and went to use the restroom when the familiar blood on the toilet paper halted my elation. I knew what was coming.

"You can come back in for another D & C tomorrow or you can wait for the miscarriage to happen naturally. I have to warn you though- at nearly thirteen weeks pregnant, this fetus will look a lot like a baby and it will be painful, like labor with strong contractions. It could take a few days for it to all be over."

I wanted to do this my way - at home with my husband, not in the operating room again. Shane and I went home and waited for the inevitable.

The doctor was right. The pain was excruciating. My husband timed the contractions and sat by my side the whole time. During the three-day ordeal, my mom helped out with Rebecca who was now in pre-Kindergarten.

At this point, we accepted that Rebecca was going to be our one and only.

Shane and I both enjoyed teaching. I was a full-time business professor at the local community college. Shane was working on his Masters to move into school administration. Life was good and we decided our family was complete.

Right after Shane's thirty-sixth birthday, I realized my irregular period was even later than usual.

I could hardly believe it when I saw that familiar plus sign. This was my fifth pregnancy and the odds were not great since only one plus sign had actually delivered a baby to my arms.

Shane and I had just begun to prioritize our marriage as Rebecca was becoming more independent. I had been consumed by motherhood when she was little, and with no discretionary income, we did not have many date nights. This unexpected pregnancy brought mixed emotions, but after a few weeks, we were on board and excited.

Throughout my pregnancy, I stayed gluten-free, and I continued to take high B12, folate and multi-vitamins. Low-dose aspirin and Lovenox were no longer recommended for MTHFR and Factor V Leiden heterozygotes (i.e. people who have only one bad copy of the gene), but I tried to keep my circulation optimal and engaged in low-intensity exercise. I was gaining far less weight with this pregnancy than I had with Rebecca. Nevertheless, my weekly check ups were reassuring, and at eighteen weeks, we found out we were having a boy!

Remington was born so early and so small that we decided we needed to call him "Remy" until he grew into his man-sized name.

Chapter 3
The Decision

I was so focused on Remy's health when he was born that I ignored my own. I started to nibble on gluten-containing foods out of sheer desperation while I was stuck in the NICU sixteen hours a day. I was pumping so frequently that I started to drink Ensure every few hours. Dairy made me break out and feel awful. Once Remy was out of the hospital, I got back on my gluten-free diet and also eliminated dairy since I suspected that both he and I were intolerant to cow's milk.

Dr. L would have certainly called me a 100 year-old by now. My thyroid hormones were bouncing all over the place. My KP had gotten bad again, and I was bloated and exhausted. We tried several different doses of Synthroid, even alternating every other day or taking a different dose once per week. Remy's medical journey aged me rapidly. I suddenly had gray hairs and wrinkles. I felt ancient.

As Remy's health improved, I realized I had put mine on hold too long. When Rebecca was little, I taught ZUMBA and did yoga three times a week. Now, I was sorely out of shape. I needed to get back into an exercise routine and figure out why I was still having so many symptoms despite being gluten-free.

When I turned thirty-nine, I started to notice pain in my joints. My hands would become stiff, my knees would hurt and my hips were as sore as they had been during my pregnancies. I feared I was developing rheumatoid arthritis, another autoimmune disease. I read that a person who has one autoimmune disease is far more likely to develop other autoimmune diseases. I did not want the one I had, let alone more!

Remy needed me to be young and energetic. Rebecca needed me to guide her through womanhood. And, I needed to have something left for myself and for Shane once the kids were grown.

I started researching (yes, this is what I do whenever I am stressed and need answers) and read about the Autoimmune Protocol (AIP), a more restricted and focused Paleo diet that targets people with autoimmune disease. I followed Dr. Izabella Wentz, read books such as *The Autoimmune Solution* by Dr. Amy Myers and *Eat Dirt* by Dr. Josh Axe, and visited incredible resources online such as thepaleomom.com, autoimmunewellness.com and aiplifestyle.com. I was convinced that AIP was for me!!

My enthusiasm was muted by the reality that this was not going to be easy. It was already difficult preparing separate meals for Remy and then modifying what I made for Shane, Rebecca and myself so that my meals were free of gluten. How was I going to swing this?

I committed to doing the strict Autoimmune Protocol for sixty days. My disciplined, organized (and a tad compulsive) personality paid off once again.

For two months, I strictly eliminated the following:
- All grains
- All dairy
- All legumes
- All nuts
- All seeds
- All refined oils
- All refined sugars
- All nightshades[32]
- Caffeine and alcohol
- Eggs
- Soy

I felt awful the first week. I had never been a drinker, so avoiding alcohol was the easy part. But, I loved chocolate and cheese (sometimes even *together*!), so I had to find recipes that were tasty and satisfying to help me

---

[32] Members of the Solanaceae family, common nightshades include white (but not sweet) potatoes, eggplant, tomatoes, and peppers, and spices such as cayenne and paprika.

forget what I was missing. I made a sweet potato and bacon hash and ate it every morning. Every. Morning.

After a week, I started to lose weight, my skin was clearing up and I began to wake up with newfound energy. Over the next two months, every symptom evaporated completely, from my sinus congestion to my numb toes.

My period arrived after twenty-eight days for the first time *in my entire life*. My hair looked fuller. I could not believe the transformation.

Then came the test...literally; I had my blood drawn pre-AIP and post-AIP, sixty days later.

Every lab improved. My thyroid antibodies[33] dropped for the first time ever. Despite eating more fats and meats, my cholesterol dropped, too. My TSH was at an ideal level without having to increase my Synthroid.

AIP is not meant to be permanent. There are certain foods that should never be reintroduced, such as gluten. However, the idea is to reset the immune system to figure out which foods cause a reaction. During the reintroduction phase, I added one food back at a time to see if I could tolerate it. After months of adding and testing my reactions, I found that the only additional foods I could tolerate were butter, white rice, and seeds.

I am still eating the sweet potato and bacon hash every morning. Every. Morning.

---

33 Hashimoto's Thyroiditis is caused by antibodies that attack the thyroid and destroy it. Most patients with Hashimoto's thyroiditis have measurable antibodies in the blood, with ~90% of patients having positive Thyroid Peroxidase (TPO) antibodies and ~50% of patients having positive Thyroglobulin Antibodies (TGA). Antibody levels can change throughout the disease course. Many patients notice a correlation between antibody level and severity of their symptoms.

BILLETTE,STEFANIE

Age 39   Collected: 07/20/2017 :08:59
Fasting: Received: 07/21/2017 :04:34
                Reported: 07/21/2017 :14:11

⚠ **THYROID PEROXIDASE AND THYROGLOBULIN ANTIBODIES**

Analyte	Value	
THYROGLOBULIN ANTIBODIES	<1	Desired Result: < or = 1 IU/mL
⚠ THYROID PEROXIDASE ANTIBODIES	173 H	Desired Result: <9 IU/mL

Performing Sites
TP Quest Diagnostics-Tampa, 4225 E Fowler Ave, Tampa, FL 33617-2026 Laboratory Director: Glen L Hortin

Key
🔵 Priority Out of Range   ⚠ Out of Range

These results have been sent to the person who ordered the tests. Your receipt of these results should not be viewed as medical advice and is not meant to replace discussion with your doctor or other healthcare professional.

Quest, Quest Diagnostics, the associated logo, Nichols Institute, Interactive Insights and all associated Quest Diagnostics marks are the registered trademarks of Quest Diagnostics. All third party marks - '®' and '™' - are the property of their respective owners. Privacy policy can be found at: http://questdiagnostics.com/home/privacy-policy/online-privacy.html. © 2020 Quest Diagnostics Incorporated. All rights reserved.

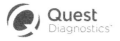

Exhibit A:
JUNE 2017 - MY THYROID PEROXIDASE ANTIBODIES WERE 173 BEFORE
AIP

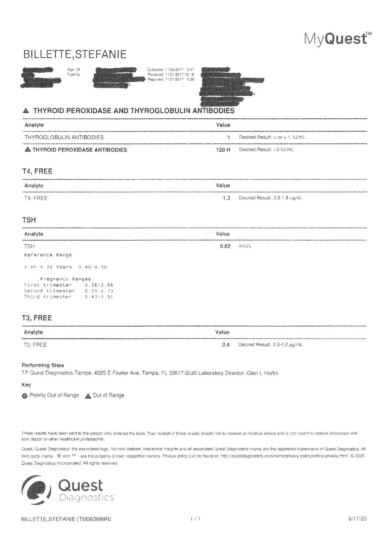

EXHIBIT B:
NOV. 2017- MY THYROID PEROXIDASE ANTIBODIES DROPPED TO 120 JUST SIXTY DAYS AFTER STARTING AIP!

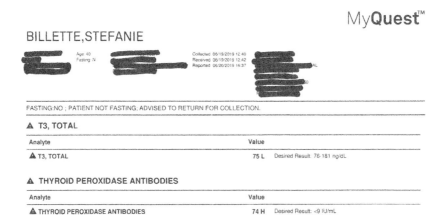

BILLETTE,STEFANIE

Age 40
Fasting: N

Collected 06/19/2019 12:40
Received 06/19/2019 12:42
Reported 06/20/2019 16:37

FASTING:NO ; PATIENT NOT FASTING. ADVISED TO RETURN FOR COLLECTION.

⚠ T3, TOTAL

Analyte	Value	
⚠ T3, TOTAL	75 L	Desired Result: 76-181 ng/dL

⚠ THYROID PEROXIDASE ANTIBODIES

Analyte	Value	
⚠ THYROID PEROXIDASE ANTIBODIES	74 H	Desired Result: <9 IU/mL

EXHIBIT C:
JUNE 2019- THYROID PEROXIDASE ANTIBODIES NEARLY TWO YEARS
LATER...
ANTIBODIES DOWN TO 74!

I fell off the AIP wagon a few times over the past three years. From August 2017 to April 2019, I did not get sick- not even when I was exposed to my son having Hand, Foot and Mouth Disease. My husband and daughter caught it from him, and I took care of all three of them. Even when my daughter caught the flu, I was spared. I suddenly felt like I had a healthy immune system.

Then, I allowed myself to start eating some non-dairy chocolate made with cocoa powder, vanilla bean and agave. What harm could it do?

Well, I got sick in April 2019. At that point, I told myself, "no more cheats".

In July 2019, both of my kids got a stomach bug. This was Remy's first virus in six months (he had not been sick since going gluten-free). I cared for them both, but I did not catch it!

A week later, for my birthday, I allowed myself some coconut milk ice cream, made with cocoa powder, vanilla bean and agave. BAM... I got sick with an upper respiratory infection. I have no doubt that the cocoa and vanilla (both legumes) as well as the refined sugar (agave) triggered inflammation and made me more vulnerable.

Then, school began. It was Remy's first year in school and my first time back in the classroom since before he was born. My diet was 99% clean, but the combination of a stressful summer moving into a new home, going back to public school teaching (middle schoolers are very germy!), being assaulted by a student, and Remy bringing home viruses from Kindergarten, was just enough to make me vulnerable.

Within six weeks of going back to the classroom, I came down with the flu. The familiar autoimmune rash emerged (very attractive, according to my hubby). But, thanks to my strict diet, I did beat the main symptoms of the flu in a just a few days with absolutely NO medication (not even ibuprofen).

The cough lingered for weeks, but it eventually went away on its own. Pre-AIP, I would have ended up on oral steroids and antibiotics.

Can I indulge and eat the wrong foods sometimes? Of course, I *can...*but I *will* pay the price, especially if I am under emotional stress. In fact, when I am under stress, even with a phenomenal diet, I can clearly become ill and have an autoimmune flare-up.

People ask me how I can be so disciplined and deprive myself of all those "yummy foods". Do I miss the foods I have given up? Of course, I do. When I make a grilled cheese sandwich for my husband, I remember how much I used to *love* eating grilled cheese sandwiches and potato chips. When we go to a restaurant and I have to spend five minutes modifying my order, do I sometimes wish I could simply order food as-is? Sure, I do!

But, then, I think about how much better I feel *not eating* those foods. I remind myself that the power I have to resist those few minutes of temptation will help me feel great later that day when I can say "I am so glad I did not give in and eat that!"

I am a very disciplined person to begin with, and after feeling sick for so many years, the choice is easy for me—a moment of pleasure followed by horrible symptoms versus moments of sheer willpower followed by a lifetime of feeling great.

I'll take the latter...any day.

STORY 3
HERS

Chapter 1
The Beginning

Rebecca was the perfect little girl. With her blond ringlets and big green eyes, she was adorable, clever and well mannered. I was often asked if I was the South American nanny since we look so different from one another.

I cherished being a mother and relished every moment with my sweet girl. Her first seven years were magical. She was identified as gifted and excelled in school. She and I were joined at the hip. My husband and I spent so much time with her that she wanted for nothing.

Despite a daily routine of brushing and flossing and a diet free of candy and sodas, she went from cavity-free at the age of three to a mouthful of decay four months later. I noticed a dark spot on one of her molars, which prompted me to take her in for an early check-up with her pediatric dentist, Dr. K, who delivered shocking news.

"Rebecca's back molars in all four quadrants have proximal caries. These are cavities between the teeth. She needs a crown and seven fillings."

After I regained my ability to speak, I asked how this could have happened. Dr. K explained that cavities are on the rise in children, and in Rebecca's case, it was likely due to many factors: her molars moved together too early, our drinking water had no fluoride (ironically, I would later buy a filtration system to get fluoride OUT of our new home's drinking water to protect Remy's liver), gummy vitamins were all the rage but can get stuck between children's teeth, and some children like Rebecca have a high concentration of strep bacteria in their saliva.

Regardless of the contributing factors, this meant extensive dental work for my munchkin. We were given two options: nitrous oxide and local anesthetics, which would require four separate visits OR intravenous sedation, which would allow completion of all the work at once. My husband and I were initially hesitant about IV sedation both because of the risks involved with this level of anesthesia and the high cost, which is usually not covered by insurance. We wanted to go with the safest plan, and all three

pediatric oral surgeons with whom I consulted said that nitrous was "completely safe".

I scheduled the first nitrous appointment. The night before the appointment, I embarked on my usual coping mechanism: research. I searched Google Scholar for medical literature on "nitrous risks" and "nitrous side effects". I came across medical studies that revealed the dangers of nitrous oxide.

Several studies illustrated a direct link between the genetic mutation MTHFR (yep, the same defect in folate metabolism that affects my B-12 level) and brain damage or even death[34]. Anyone low in vitamin B-12 (e.g. some vegetarians or vegans) can have adverse outcomes to nitrous oxide exposure[35]. There is much research that shows nitrous oxide can be neurotoxic, especially after repeated exposure.

The neurological effects from nitrous have led to its overuse and abuse as a recreational drug. For this reason, nitrous oxide has been banned in dental practices in most European countries and there is current pressure in the U.S. to ban its sale completely.

I canceled Rebecca's appointment and, after an unsuccessful attempt to treat her using Novocaine alone, she underwent IV sedation without the use of nitrous. I educated her dentist and anesthesiologist about nitrous oxide risks. They were surprised and appreciated having this new information.

Children are not routinely screened for metabolic disorders or for vitamin deficiencies. Yet, nitrous is routinely used in pediatric dental offices across the United States. "Laughing gas" may sound innocuous, but the research shows how risky it can be if a child has an underlying condition or a diet that depletes them of Vitamin B-12. Ask questions, demand blood

[34] https://www.ncbi.nlm.nih.gov/pmc/articles/PMC5932993/
[35] https://www.ncbi.nlm.nih.gov/pmc/articles/PMC4066238/

work, and don't let anyone minimize your fears by saying the risk is only "one in a million". You or your child may just be that one.

Chapter 2
The Choice

A few more years passed, and we were happily living as a trio. When I became pregnant and lost the baby, we lit a candle and shed a tear. Then, when Rebecca was six, we told her we were pregnant again and she was thrilled. When Remy was born, she handled the change like a trooper...at first.

She adored her little brother, but she resented the time he took away from her. She missed one-on-one time with me and she missed being the sole star and focus of her family.

As she approached her pre-teens and Remy's health improved, I started to notice some familiar symptoms. She was bloated, gaining weight in her abdomen, she was developing KP on her arms and legs, she was starting to get acne, she was often down in the dumps, she had low energy, and she slept a lot. Her growth had also slowed.

"Mommy, why am I so tired? I haven't done anything today?" Rebecca implored.

I decided to take her to a pediatric endocrinologist and explained my concerns. Much like myself at her age, Rebecca was addicted to carbs. I told the endocrinologist about her love of sweets.

I had always been a savvy grocery shopper, avoiding high fructose corn syrup and hydrogenated oils and buying organic and non-GMO foods for my family. But, even organic, non-GMO cookies have sugar and Rebecca would eat a dozen if I let her. And, unlike me, she did not love the vegetables and proteins I would prepare from scratch each evening. I make a Persian stew with lots of greens and meat that she loves to eat, but she would always eat the rice before the protein and veggies. Even worse, Rebecca was not as motivated as I have always been to exercise and get fit.

Dr. B agreed to test her for celiac, diabetes, and thyroid disease. Her insulin came back high, but she did not have diabetes, although Dr. B said she could be on the road to Type 2 Diabetes if she didn't cut back on sugar. She tested negative for celiac (like me). But, her thyroid antibodies were elevated and her Thyroid Stimulating Hormone (TSH) was 4.34. Her high antibodies confirmed what I suspected. She had Hashimoto's Autoimmune Thyroid disease.

If there are low levels of thyroid hormone circulating in the bloodstream, then the pituitary gland produces TSH, which stimulates the thyroid gland to manufacture and secrete more thyroid hormones (T3 and T4). Therefore, high TSH levels indicate that there is not enough T3 and T4 in the bloodstream, which results from an underactive thyroid. I have long known that a TSH value between 3 and 4, while accepted by labs and physicians as within "normal range" is not ideal or healthy. It took me years to realize that I felt my best when my TSH was around 1-1.5.

"Rebecca, I don't want you to go through the decades of torment I experienced".

"I'm only eleven! I don't want to go AIP. I love chocolate!" Rebecca started to cry.

"Listen, honey. If you eliminate gluten now, I am very confident you will never have to go full AIP."

It took a lot of cajoling and convincing, but she agreed that she would go gluten-free. I told her she would feel better, look healthier and her labs would improve. I promised her that we were doing the right thing.

Chapter 3
The Proof

Within a few weeks, Rebecca's bloating and stomach cramping subsided. Her acne improved. Most importantly, her energy and mood were noticeably better.

When we went in for the follow-up labs, I was pleased but unsurprised. Her TSH had dropped to 1.5!

When we saw Dr. B, I beamed. "The only change we made since the first set of labs was the elimination of gluten!"

Like many doctors, she seemed impressed but skeptical as to why this would have worked.

"Well, I don't know why it helped, but it can't hurt to keep her gluten free."

Most doctors think if a patient is not celiac, then there is no issue with gluten. Most medical practitioners poorly understand non-celiac gluten sensitivity[36]. What they fail to realize is that gluten triggers inflammation in people with autoimmune disease and creates a cascade of negative reactions within the body, including fatigue, bloating, brain fog and joint pain.[37]

After five months on a gluten-free diet, Rebecca's antibodies started to drop! Rebecca is now twelve and her health has improved dramatically. She doesn't get sick as often as she used to and is not depressed anymore. Her

---

[36] https://celiac.org/about-celiac-disease/related-conditions/non-celiac-wheat-gluten-sensitivity/

[37] https://www.beyondceliac.org/celiac-disease/non-celiac-gluten-sensitivity/what-is-it/

body is now growing and developing as it was intended, before autoimmune disease tried to rob her of wellness.

Looking back at her blood work, I see that in 2017 her thyroid antibodies were normal, but her growth was slowing. In February 2019, her labs revealed Hashimoto's Thyroiditis (the same autoimmune disease that my mother and I have). What triggered her autoimmune disease is a mystery. For me, it was likely mono. For her, the genetic predisposition was so strong that perhaps the trigger was multiple rounds of antibiotics for frequent ear infections as an infant. Perhaps her trigger was the flu from the year prior.

We may never know the exact trigger, and there may not have been just one. As with Remy, it would be nice to know *why*, but I will take a treatment that works over knowing *why* any day.

Although her thyroid is still being attacked by autoantibodies (antibodies against "the self"), Rebecca's thyroid gland is now saying "Bring it on; I am still going to do my job". When she was eating gluten, her thyroid laid down, much like she did, and said "I am too tired; do whatever you want."

I often wonder what would have happened if my own experiences had not primed me to recognize the symptoms of autoimmune thyroid disease. Rebecca likely would have continued down a road of fatigue, depression, weight gain, and hormonal imbalances. I am grateful that my journey allowed me to identify her disease early.

I wish she did not have to deal with it at all. But, unfortunately, more people (especially women) are being diagnosed with Hashimoto's and other autoimmune disorders. Genetics, our food supply and environmental toxins all play a role in this alarming trend. But, until doctors recognize the symptoms of autoimmune diseases and acknowledge that food is a key component to managing these conditions, we will always have to play both patient and physician for our loved ones and ourselves.

BILLETTE, REBECCA

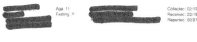

Age: 11
Fasting: Y

Collected: 02/19/2019 06:52
Received: 02/19/2019 06:53
Reported: 02/27/2019 19:05

FASTING:YES ; MULTIPLE TESTING PRIORITIES; ROUTINE TESTING TO FOLLOW.

▲ TSH

Analyte	Value
▲ TSH	4.34 H mIU/L

Reference Range

1-19 Years 0.50-4.30

Pregnancy Ranges
First trimester   0.26-2.66
Second trimester 0.55-2.73
Third trimester   0.43-2.91

▲ T4, FREE

Analyte	Value
▲ T4, FREE	1.5 H Desired Result: 0.9-1.4 ng/dL

▲ THYROID PEROXIDASE AND THYROGLOBULIN ANTIBODIES

Analyte	Value
▲ THYROGLOBULIN ANTIBODIES	11 H Desired Result: < or = 1 IU/mL
THYROID PEROXIDASE ANTIBODIES	1 Desired Result: <9 IU/mL

EXHIBIT E:
FEB. 2019- REBECCA'S HIGH TSH PRE- GLUTEN-FREE (4.34) AND HIGH THYROGLOBULIN ANTIBODIES (11)

MyQuest™

BILLETTE,REBECCA R

  Age: 11
Fasting: N
Collected: 05/17/2019 08:26
Received: 05/17/2019 08:28
Reported: 05/20/2019 16:05

FASTING:NO

⚠ **THYROID PEROXIDASE AND THYROGLOBULIN ANTIBODIES**

Analyte	Value	
⚠ THYROGLOBULIN ANTIBODIES	44 H	Desired Result: < or = 1 IU/mL
THYROID PEROXIDASE ANTIBODIES	3	Desired Result: <9 IU/mL

TSH

Analyte	Value	
TSH	1.84	mIU/L

Reference Range

1-19 Years 0.50-4.30

Pregnancy Ranges
First trimester 0.26-2.66
Second trimester 0.55-2.73
Third trimester 0.43-2.91

T4 (THYROXINE), TOTAL

Analyte	Value	
T4 (THYROXINE), TOTAL	7.0	Desired Result: 5.7-11.6 mcg/dL

T4, FREE

Analyte	Value	
T4, FREE	1.1	Desired Result: 0.9-1.4 ng/dL

Performing Sites
TP Quest Diagnostics-Tampa, 4225 E Fowler Ave, Tampa, FL 33617-2026 Laboratory Director: Glen L Hortin

Key
🔵 Priority Out of Range   ⚠ Out of Range

EXHIBIT F:
MAY 2019- REBECCA'S TSH IS MUCH BETTER AFTER THREE MONTHS
GLUTEN FREE (1.84)
HIGH THYROGLOBULIN ANTIBODIES (44)

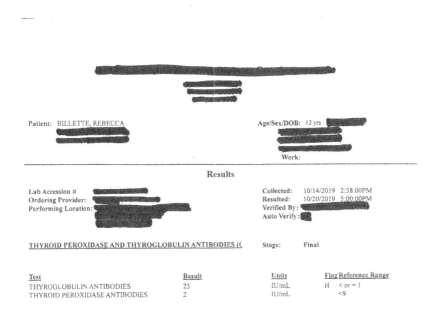

Patient: BILLETTE, REBECCA   Age/Sex/DOB: 12 yrs

                                                      Work:

Results

Lab Accession #   Collected: 10/14/2019 2:38:00PM
Ordering Provider: Resulted: 10/20/2019 5:00:00PM
Performing Location: Verified By:
                                                      Auto Verify:

THYROID PEROXIDASE AND THYROGLOBULIN ANTIBODIES (C   Stage: Final

Test	Result	Units	Flag	Reference Range
THYROGLOBULIN ANTIBODIES	23	IU/mL	H	< or = 1
THYROID PEROXIDASE ANTIBODIES	2	IU/mL		<9

EXHIBIT G:
OCT. 2019 -REBECCA'S THYROGLOBULIN ANTIBODIES BEGAN DROPPING NINE MONTHS AFTER GOING GLUTEN-FREE (23)!

STORY 4
YOURS

Chapter 1
The Truth

You have heard it all.

"Big Belly?"
"Don't eat wheat!"

"Brain Fog?"
"Don't eat grains!"

"Low energy?"
"Go Paleo!"

"Want to prevent cancer?"
"Don't eat red meat!"

"Want to lose weight?"
"Go Vegan!"

All of these diets and protocols profess to have the answer. They all claim:

"This. Is. The. Diet. For. Everyone."

Here is the truth. EVERYONE has SOMETHING that they should stop eating, which will lead to improved health. It may be as simple as eliminating coffee so that you can avoid that 10 a.m. attack of heartburn. Or maybe you notice that every time you eat beans, you get bloated and have stomach pain. Chances are that you already *know* which foods give you problems. And, perhaps that is why you picked up this book. Maybe you were curious about the title. Maybe you realized that all the fad diets you have tried don't address your specific condition.

I am not telling you to eliminate everything. For some, like me, there are many foods that had to be eliminated to feel well again. Hopefully, my daughter only needed to eliminate gluten. For my son, he had to eliminate many foods in order to survive.

I used to be judgmental (OK, I still am to a degree). I used to think when children had meltdowns, it was all the parents' fault. I used to think since my daughter was well behaved it was only because I was a good mom. Having Remy taught me that there are so many factors that go into a child's early development. Living in a plastic box and fighting for one's life does affect behavior and temperament. Going from an only child for six years to having to give up the spotlight for an ill sibling does affect a child's anxiety level and coping skills.

Diet can have a profound effect on anger, patience, and mood for both children and their parents. Very few physicians and psychologists will ever ask a patient about his/her diet. As a former teacher, I could tell you the moment my students walked into my classroom who among them had a nutritious breakfast and who grabbed a pack of Doritos and chocolate milk on the way out the door. I had many students who were labeled ADD/ADHD and regularly ate candies laden with food colorings, such as red dye 40, which has been shown to negatively affect cognition and behavior, exacerbating (if not directly creating) ADD/ADHD symptoms[38]. Sadly, most parents look to pharmaceuticals to control ADD/ADHD symptoms instead of looking in their pantries.

It is important to eat nutritious foods, but it is equally, if not more essential, to *avoid* eating foods that harm the body. Food additives, such as dyes and chemicals are doubly detrimental since they not only deprive you of vital vitamins and minerals, but they also work against your body as it tries to absorb nutrients.

[38] https://www.ncbi.nlm.nih.gov/pmc/articles/PMC3441937/

It is easier in the short term to feed your body what is quick and convenient. But, it will take much more time and energy in the long haul to manage the chronic diseases that follow. Beyond metabolic and autoimmune diseases, there are many conditions that can affect your quality of life and are preventable. Type 1 Diabetes is an autoimmune disease that has a strong genetic component, and it usually presents in childhood. Type 2 Diabetes usually occurs later in life, but recently it has been on the rise, caused primarily by lifestyle factors, and patients are getting diagnosed younger and younger.[39] Lifestyle factors include high blood pressure, overweight or obesity, insufficient physical activity, poor diet, and fat stored in the waist.

The definition of poor diet is where most misunderstanding and misinformation begins. What is *poor* diet? Too much meat? Too much fat? Not enough vegetables?

Most functional physicians, many nurse practitioners and a great number of health coaches, like myself, have reviewed the data and seen the results. The one commonality that drives a poor diet is *excess sugar*.

When people think of "obese", they usually associate it with eating too much fat. But, fat is not the enemy. Healthy fats such as unrefined oils and avocados are nutritious and have numerous health benefits. But, instead of eating healthy fats, many people count calories and fall for the "diet soda" or "low-fat food" craze.

At best, artificial sweeteners can make you consume a high quantity of foods with low nutritive value, and worse, they can contribute to metabolic disorders.[40] Low-fat or no-fat dairy does not have the right ratios of protein and fats so they need additives and fillers to give them the right texture. If you are going to eat dairy, it is far better to have a small serving of "real" ice cream rather than a pint of sugar-free low-fat ice cream.

[39] https://www.nih.gov/news-events/news-releases/rates-new-diagnosed-cases-type-1-type-2-diabetes-rise-among-children-teens
[40] https://www.health.harvard.edu/blog/artificial-sweeteners-sugar-free-but-at-what-cost-201207165030

You Are What You *DON'T* Eat

Many people add refined sugar to their coffee and eat deserts regularly. In fact, it is the consumption of sugar (not *fat*) that leads to fatty liver[41]. When Remy was in the NICU, he developed fatty liver, not because of my breast milk, but because of the sucrose he was being given regularly. While Remy has a specific mutation that inhibits the breakdown of fructose, even people without an inherited error of metabolism can overload their livers with sugars. Much like with alcoholism, sugar addiction will destroy hepatic cells over time and lead to liver disease[42].

Some people avoid "sweets" such as cookies and cakes but instead eat high amounts of fruits. While fruit has many vitamins and minerals, eating too much fruit means eating too much fructose. Fructose is the only sugar that is completely metabolized by the liver. Too much of it can cause fatty liver, insulin resistance and other complications, so be kind to your liver and limit sugar- in all its forms.[43]

[41]
https://www.ncbi.nlm.nih.gov/pmc/articles/PMC4405421/#:~:text=Increased%20consumption%20of%20sugar%2Dsweetened%20beverages%20and%20pre%2Dpackaged%20foods, %26%20nonalcoholic%20steatohepatitis%20(NASH).

[42] https://www.sciencedaily.com/releases/2020/06/200629120250.htm

[43] https://www.health.harvard.edu/heart-health/abundance-of-fructose-not-good-for-the-liver-heart

Chapter 2

The Power

The concept of the elimination diet was first proposed by Dr. Albert Rowe in 1926 and elucidated in his book, *Elimination Diets and the Patient's Allergies*, published in 1944.

Yet, the role that is played by dietary factors in the pathogenesis and progression of disease is only now being taken seriously. For years, western medicine focused on pharmaceuticals to cure every ailment. Instead of looking for the root cause of symptoms, most physicians preferred to give patients a pill. The problem is that one pill can cause a host of other problems sending patients right back to the doctor with more symptoms. This is how some people end up taking dozens of medications each day and still don't feel well. Over the past decade, many physicians are taking a functional approach to medicine, seeking to heal through diet and lifestyle factors instead of prescription drugs.

It took years for Remy and I to find our "safe" and "unsafe" food lists. Here is a breakdown of the foods we each eat on a daily basis. There is some overlap, but there are also key differences.

Remy's Diet	Stefanie's Diet
+meat and fish	+meat and fish
+olive oil, ghee, butter	+olive oil, ghee, butter
+ white rice/oat/tapioca/corn starch	+white Rice/root veggies and their flours/tapioca flour
+dairy	+non-nightshade veggies
+plain coffee (when he is older)	+fruits (limit)
+dark greens (stalks removed)	+herbs
+herbs	+maple syrup and honey
+eggs	+coconut products
Absolutely NO: fruits, vegetables, soy, nuts, legumes, seeds, spices, wheat,	Absolutely NO: soy, dairy, grains, legumes, nuts or nut oils,

brown rice, sweet potatoes, sweeteners of any kind (natural or artificial), alcohol, or chocolate.	nightshade veggies and spices, sweeteners (natural or artificial), chocolate, alcohol, eggs

Based on the table above, you can surmise several facts:

1. Our grocery bills are high
2. We don't go out to dinner often
3. We only travel to places where I have access to a full kitchen
4. I cook for several hours each day
5. We own a lot of coolers and ice packs

Medical diets are different from fad diets. Fad diets are usually aimed at weight loss. Medical diets are necessary in order to move from disease to wellness. When you know how badly you feel as a result of eating certain foods and how great you feel when you eliminate them, it does not feel like much of a sacrifice. It is like looking at a non-edible item like your cell phone and thinking "Um, why would I want to eat that? It's not food to *me*!"

When we discovered Remy couldn't metabolize fructose, my husband made the choice to show solidarity with our son. He decided to never eat sweets or fruits again. It has been nearly fours years since he made that promise and Remy is always excited to say, "Daddy and I don't eat cookies and cakes". He is not alone. My husband recently decided to eliminate gluten as well. He has had digestive issues for years and hopes this change will help alleviate his gastrointestinal distress. I know it will help; the question is whether it will help enough.

If you have been diagnosed with Hashimoto's, Crohn's, or any other autoimmune disease and your physician tells you that diet does not matter, find a new doctor! This happened to my friend whose gastroenterologist told her to take a pill every day to control her Crohn's symptoms. She asked if it may help her to modify her diet, and he said, "No, diet doesn't matter. Just take the pill every day. That is all you need to do". Her instincts told her otherwise. I encouraged her to start by eliminating gluten. Her symptoms finally started to improve after two months gluten-free.

I have found many amazing recipes online, some fructose-free, others gluten-free, many autoimmune-friendly. I have had to tweak, modify and sometimes downright invent many of my go-to recipes. I share many of these with you at the end of this book. You can also find posts, recipes and other information on my blog. [44]

Each of our diets is different, so I have to find the common threads to create a core meal (protein) and then add veggies (for all of us but Remy) and then a carb we can all have (basmati rice or rice noodles). For breakfast, we all eat bacon. My son has oatmeal, I have a sweet potato and my daughter and husband have gluten-free toast (I make our breads in a bread machine).

For lunch, I pack meat sticks, berries and plantain chips for myself. Rebecca has snacks like popcorn, cheese, and apples. Remy eats my homemade oat crackers and homemade hamburger patties or meatballs. Shane usually grabs tacos. When we travel (which we don't do often), we get accommodations with a full kitchen. We don't eat out much, but if we do, we look for restaurants that are very accommodating and will modify meals.

You are not helpless. There is power in knowledge and in making choices. I don't like the term "restricted diet" because it sounds like you have to give up something that is good for you and suffer.

Support is the key as you navigate your path to healing through dietary change. While we are all on different diets, tailored to heal our unique bodies, my husband, daughter, son, and I support each other. Your family should celebrate your health – even if, at times, it makes things inconvenient.

[44] www.TakeBackYourBody.com/blog

Elimination diets put you in control. By eliminating problem foods, you will see that the most important decisions you make will revolve around what you *don't* put in your mouth. Therein lies your power over illness.

Chapter 3
The Future

If you have an autoimmune disease, you can start by eliminating gluten and see how your health improves. If it is not enough, you may need to go further down the elimination path.

I know what you're thinking. "Why give up everything? I will just give up one food at a time and see which one is causing my issues!"

That may work for an eleven year-old like my daughter who was at the very beginning of her disease course, but it may not help someone who has battled autoimmune symptoms for years. It is much easier to detect sensitivities by eliminating all inflammatory foods at once and then adding *one food back at a time*. Think about how we introduce foods to an infant. Can you imagine if we gave an infant all fruits, grains, and veggies at once and then asked, "I wonder which one is causing that rash?"

Food should nourish, not poison. Find out what triggers YOUR symptoms and eliminate it. If you have inflammation of any kind, treat it as an autoimmune condition, because if you don't treat it now, it may become one at some point in your life.

If you have eliminated gluten and your symptoms have not improved, I suggest following my AIM: *Auto*Immune *M*ethod to Take Back Your Body[45]. My method focuses on three components: dietary, stress, and support. Each of these is vital to achieving and maintaining the quality of life that you deserve.

You can still enjoy delicious meals. You can still socialize. You can still enjoy life. My recipes can help you plan and prep meals that are easy and satisfying.

---

[45] https://www.takebackyourbody.com/stefanies-autoimmune-method

Resist the urge to "cheat" as you will feel the effects afterward. It may be bloating if you are gluten-sensitive, or it may be arthritic joints if you have Hashimoto's and decide to eat a tomato. It may be subtle or short-lived, but your "small cheat" will have an effect. On the other hand, forgive yourself if you do have a cheat. You *can* restart and *will* reset.

I encourage you to get labs done before you embark on this life-changing journey and then get labs again after sixty days. You will be amazed by the changes you will see. And, you will be thrilled with the changes you will feel!

The social and cultural aspects of eating are powerful. But, so are you. Nevertheless, sometimes it is easier to embark on life-changing endeavors with a bit of help. Certified Health Coaches, like myself, help others feel their best through individualized food and lifestyle changes that meet their unique needs and health goals.

I hope this book has inspired you to find out what you should *not* be eating so that you can enjoy what you do eat and start living.

Remy, enjoying a homemade saffron popsicle

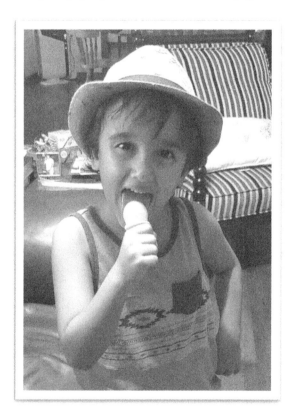

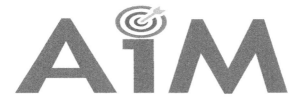

AutoImmune Method

I created the AIM: Autoimmune Method which echoes the main tenets of the Autoimmune Protocol (AIP); however, I added to AIP by incorporating my own research and experience to create a triad of healing. My AIM: AutoImmune Method has three components, each essential to autoimmune healing.

THE DIETARY COMPONENT

FOR THE FIRST 60 DAYS, AVOID:

DAIRY   EGGS   GRAINS   NIGHTSHADES (INCLUDES EGGPLANT, WHITE POTATO, TOMATO, AND NIGHTSHADE SPICES SUCH AS CAYENNE, CHILI, PAPRIKA)   LEGUMES   GUMS   NUTS   ARTIFICIAL SWEETENERS   SEEDS   EMULSIFIERS   CAFFEINE   FOOD THICKENERS   ALCOHOL   NSAIDS (INCLUDES IBUPROFEN) REFINED OR PROCESSED FOODS   ARTIFICIAL COLORS AND FLAVORINGS REFINED SUGAR   CHEMICAL ADDITIVES   REFINED OILS   TRANS FATS   PSEUDOGRAINS

BUT, YOU CAN ENJOY:

COCONUT PRODUCTS (ESPECIALLY OILS AND MILK) RED MEAT (MOSTLY LEAN AND PREFERABLY GRASS-FED, BUT AT LEAST ORGANIC)   OLIVE OIL   POULTRY AND PORK (PASTURE-RAISED)   GHEE   SEAFOOD FERMENTED FOODS   VEGETABLES (INCLUDING ROOT VEGGIES SUCH AS SWEET POTATO)   VINEGARS   BERRIES   HONEY   HERBAL TEAS MAPLE SYRUP   HERBS   ARROWROOT, CASSAVA, TAPIOCA, AND COCONUT FLOURS   ORGAN MEATS   AVOCADO OIL   SEA SALT BLACK PEPPER

You don't have to feel deprived. You just have to plan and prepare!

I order most of my meats and fish from ButcherBox.com and grasslandbeef.com. Every day, I go to my deep freezer and decide what I will need to make the following day. I place those items in my refrigerator. I buy fresh organic produce every few days and have a full supply of all my essential flours and starches in my pantry. Planning ahead gives me control and therefore eases my stress when it comes to meal preparation. I spend about 2-3 hours each day preparing meals and snacks for my family, and there is nothing that gives me more satisfaction than knowing I am giving them healing and nutritious foods.

THE STRESS COMPONENT

Your diet can be ideal, but without stress management, you will not heal completely.

SLEEP:

Pick a consistent bedtime and wake-time that will give you at least 8 hours of sleep per night. Avoid napping since it will interfere with your circadian rhythm. Unless you are ill, the need to nap is a sign that you are not resting enough at night.

We have all met people who say they don't need 8 hours of sleep. We can all "make it work" in the short term, but the long-term immunological effects of inadequate sleep are just now being recognized. Get your rest and your body will be better prepared for whatever challenges it faces.

EXERCISE:

You should engage in at least 30 minutes of moderate-intensity exercise most days of the week (e.g. walking, jogging, Pilates, swimming, singles tennis). You also want to engage in weight-bearing exercise 3-5 times per week. Women are especially vulnerable to osteoporosis, particularly if you take synthetic hormone replacement.

RELAXATION/DETOX:

Essential oils have been shown to reduce anxiety and stress, which has a beneficial effect on one's immune response.[46] As a certified holistic aromatherapist, I make blends for my family that ease the stress load and encourage a positive immune response.

---

[46] https://www.ncbi.nlm.nih.gov/pmc/articles/PMC1142199/

It is also imperative to avoid environmental toxins as much as possible. I recommend a HEPA air purifier in every room of your house, avoid purchasing any products that contain vinyl since they emit dangerous VOCs (volatile organic compounds) and avoid personal care products that contain common hormonal disruptors, such as: aluminum, parabens, phthalates, dioxin, and BPA. Never use antiperspirant (these products clog lymph nodes close to the breast and may contribute to breast cancer). My daughter and I use natural deodorant instead.[47]

THE SUPPORT COMPONENT

In order to be successful, you will need support from friends and family. It is important that your relationships help you during this period of change instead of hindering your progress. You must maintain healthy and enriching relationships and rid yourself of toxic and negative relationships. This includes both personal relationships and professional ones.

You may also need supplements, which will support your body as it heals.

My personal belief is that some multivitamins cause more harm than good. I have found a multivitamin[48] that has high quality forms of each essential vitamin and mineral (e.g. methylated B12) and does not over-supply the body. If you are on a limited diet, it is likely you are missing some key vitamins or minerals, so a minimalistic multi-vitamin may be a good idea.

[47] https://www.amazon.com/Alvera-Natural-Roll-Deodorant-Almonds/dp/B0014AY7M2

[48] https://www.thorne.com/products/dp/basic-nutrients-2-day-vm2nc

Many of us (especially those of us with sluggish thyroids) are very deficient in Vitamin D (whether this is a cause or an effect is up for debate). Low vitamin D has been linked to chronic constipation and other symptoms[49]. Experts agree that

adults can take up to 4000 IU of Vitamin D daily to prevent infections and immune system disorders.[50]

Finally, I highly recommend that you not only learn how to prepare the majority of your meals from scratch, but learn how to grow your own food, too!

My children and I recently started growing our own microgreens.[51] Microgreens grow quickly, take minimal space and have a delicate flavor due to their small size. It is incredibly satisfying to plant, nurture, harvest and consume food that you have created yourself (almost as if that is what we were meant to do...)!

[49] https://www.ncbi.nlm.nih.gov/pmc/articles/PMC6465937/

[50] https://my.clevelandclinic.org/health/articles/15050-vitamin-d--vitamin-d-deficiency

[51] https://wellnessmama.com/36688/grow-microgreens/

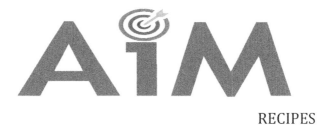

RECIPES

These are a few of the recipes I have created. They require minimal ingredients and prep time. To see my recipes in full-color, visit my blog: www.takebackyourbody.com/blog

Stefanie's AIM: AutoImmune Method Sweet Potato Hash (cast iron skillet)

Ingredients:

12 oz. bacon (I recommend Maverick No Sugar or grasslandbeef.com bacon) cut into 1-inch pieces
2 TBSP Ghee or Coconut Oil
4 cups diced zucchini or celery
6 cups diced sweet potatoes
1 cup chopped yellow onion
Salt and Black Pepper To Taste

Directions:

1. In a cast iron skillet, cook bacon pieces over med-low heat until crisp
2. Remove cooked bacon using a slotted spoon. Add coconut oil or ghee to the skillet.
3. Pre-heat oven to 400 degrees F.
4. Fry the sweet potatoes in the skillet on med-high heat until they are golden-brown and start to soften.
5. Add zucchini/celery and onion and cook until they begin to soften.
6. Stir in bacon and remove from heat.
7. Place skillet in the oven and bake 30 minutes.
8. You can top this with Mastodon AIP Sauce by KC Natural

Stefanie's AIM: AutoImmune Method "Pita Bread"

Ingredients:

½ cup Cassava Flour (I use Otto's)
½ cup Tapioca Flour (I use Bob's Red Mill)
¼ tsp. sesame seeds (if you have completed the first sixty days and successfully added seeds back into your diet)
3 TBSP Salted Butter or Ghee (grass-fed)
¾ cup filtered water
¼ tsp. sea salt

Directions:

1. Pre-heat oven to 400 degrees F.
2. Mix all ingredients together in a large bowl.
3. Pour the mixture onto unbleached parchment paper (I use "If you care").
4. Spread the mixture to about 1/8 inch thickness across the parchment paper.
5. Bake for 20-25 minutes until crispy. Eat as a "pita" or break apart into "crackers".

Stefanie's AIM: AutoImmune Method "Best Salad Ever"

Ingredients*:

Romaine Lettuce
Sliced cucumber
Sliced white mushrooms
Sunflower Seeds (after initial 60 days- if you have been able to ad them back in without reaction)
Chopped Red cabbage
Sliced Carrots
Sliced Heart of Palm

*Add as much as you want of each

Dressing:

3 tbsp. lemon juice
3 tbsp. olive oil
1 tbsp. coconut milk
1 tbsp. apple cider vinegar
¼ tsp. dried dill
½ tsp. sea salt

Stefanie's AIM: Autoimmune Method Coconut Maple Lime Popsicles

Ingredients:

Coconut Milk (I use Thai Kitchen)
Maple Syrup (I use 365 or Trader Joe's Pure Maple Syrup)
Fresh Limes

Directions:

1. Using a silicone Popsicle mold, fill the mold halfway with coconut milk.
2. Then, pour a few drops of maple syrup into the mold (adjust quantity depending on the size of your mold).
3. Squeeze half a lime into the mold (you may want to a whole lime if you like lime a lot like I do!)
4. Freeze until solid.

Stefanie's AIM: Autoimmune Method "Sweet Bread"

Ingredients:

1-½ cups of coconut milk
¼ butter
2 TBSP unsweetened applesauce
¼ cup honey
1 tsp. apple cider vinegar
1/3 cup salted butter
1 cup each of the following flours: white rice flour, cassava flour, and tapioca flour
1 tsp. sea salt
1 packet of Red Star gluten-free yeast

Directions:

1. Add wet ingredients to bread machine
2. Add dry ingredients (except yeast) to bread machine.
3. Make a hole in the center and add yeast.
4. Set machine to gluten-free setting

Stefanie's AIM: Autoimmune Method Pot Roast

Ingredients:

2 lb. Grass-Fed Chuck Roast (I order mine from grasslandbeef.com)
2 Organic Zucchini
2 Organic Squash
1 Organic Yellow Onion
2 Turnips
$\frac{1}{2}$ tbsp. ground ginger
$\frac{1}{2}$ tbsp. turmeric
$\frac{1}{2}$ tbsp. sea salt
$\frac{1}{2}$ tbsp. garlic powder

Directions:
1. Add sliced zucchini, squash, onion to slow-cooker (I use a clay pot slow cooker)
2. Then, add cubed turnips
3. Add all spices/seasonings
4. Add water to cover the vegetables
5. Add chuck roast
6. Cook on "stew" for a minimum of 4 hours to ensure that the meat falls apart

Stefanie's Fructose-Free Parm Crisps with Oregano (safe for HFI/not for those with autoimmune diseases)

Ingredients:

Shredded non-GMO Parmesan Cheese
Olive oil
Organic Dried Oregano
Sea Salt

Directions:

1. On a microwave-safe plate, place a piece of unbleached parchment paper.
2. Make 6 mounds on the plate, each with one heaping tablespoon of shredded Parmesan cheese
3. Sprinkle ¼ tsp. of sea salt evenly among the 6 mounds
4. Drizzle 1 tsp. of olive oil evenly among the 6 mounds
5. Sprinkle 1/4 tsp. oregano evenly among the 6 mounds
6. Place the plate in the microwave for one minute
7. Remove plate from microwave and place in the refrigerator for 5 minutes

Stefanie's AIM: Autoimmune Method Parfait

Ingredients:

Raw and unsalted sunflower seeds
Raspberries and blackberries
Full-fat coconut milk

Directions:

1. Fill an ice cream cup with ½ cup of coconut milk.
2. Add ½ cup of fresh raspberries and blackberries
3. Add 1 tbsp. of sunflower seeds (if you have been able to add sunflower seeds back into your diet after your 60-day AIM reset)

Stefanie's Fructose-Free and Gluten-Free "Rice Cookies" (safe for HFI/ not for those with autoimmune diseases during the 60-day reset)

Ingredients:

½ cup of granulated rice
1/3 cup salted butter
1 egg yolk
1 TBSP tapioca dextrose (I buy Mike's Tapioca Dextrose)

Directions:

1. Preheat oven to 350 degrees.
2. Mix cream of rice and tapioca dextrose in a small bowl.
3. Mix melted butter and egg yolk in another small bowl.
4. Combine wet and dry ingredients.
5. Mold mixture into "domes" so that they are thicker in the middle (this will create for crispy edges).
6. Bake for 18 minutes.

Stefanie's Gluten-Free Fructose-Free Waffles (safe for HFI/ not for those with autoimmune diseases)

Ingredients:

1/2 cup gluten-free white rice flour
$\frac{1}{2}$ cup gluten-free tapioca flour
$\frac{1}{2}$ cup gluten-free cornstarch
$\frac{1}{2}$ cup gluten-free oat flour
$\frac{1}{2}$ teaspoon sea salt
$\frac{1}{2}$ tsp. xanthan gum
6 tbsp. ghee or safflower oil
2 large eggs
1 tbsp. gluten-free baking powder
1-$\frac{1}{2}$ cups of oat milk

Directions:

1. Mix all dry ingredients. Mix all wet ingredients.
2. Whisk the wet and dry together.
3. Pour into waffle maker. Makes 3-4 waffles.

Stefanie's AIM: Autoimmune Method Ice Cream

Ingredients:

4 cups Full-fat coconut milk
½ tbsp. Rosewater
1 tsp. Maple Syrup

Directions:

Using an ice cream maker, pour all ingredients into the frozen bowl and churn for 30 minutes.

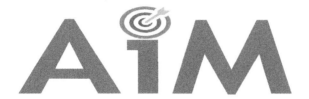

Essential Oil Blends

As a certified NAHA Level 1 Holistic Aromatherapist, I have studied the science behind essential oils. This is not voo-doo. The medicines we use today originated in plants, which have since been patented for profit. Plant-based healing is powerful. Essential oils are effective both aromatically and topically. Migraines, congestion and many other symptoms can improve with the right blend.

Stefanie's AIM: AutoImmune Method "Protection" Custom Blend

Ingredients:

2 drops of Eucalyptus Globulus Essential Oil

2 drops of Lemon Essential Oil

1 drop of Oregano Essential Oil

Directions:

You can 3-5 drops of this blend to your diffuser along with filtered water.

This blend highlights the antiviral properties of Oregano, the cleansing properties of Lemon, and the camphorous properties of Eucalyptus while creating a pleasant aroma. I regularly inhale this blend. It kept me from getting sick when everyone in my house was ill with Hand, Foot and Mouth. I boil water, pour into a mug, and place these oils in the mug. I put a towel over my head and inhale the steam for 3-5 minutes twice daily.

Stefanie's AIM: AutoImmune Method "Clarity" Custom Blend

Ingredients:

2 drops of Ylang Ylang Essential Oil

2 drops of Lemon Essential Oil

1 drop of Peppermint Essential Oil (do not use in presence of children under the age of 10)

Directions:

You can 3-5 drops of this blend to your diffuser along with filtered water.

This blend can be diffused in every room of your home to clean the air and invigorate your mind.

Thank you for reading *You Are What You DON'T Eat.* If you enjoyed and learned from this book, please recommend it to others who need it. I appreciate reviews on Amazon as well as visits and subscriptions to my blog and YouTube channel!

www.TakeBackYourBody.com/blog

ACKNOWLEDGEMENTS

Thank you to my husband, Shane, for putting our family above all else.

Thank you to my mom, Jennifer, for being with me during the hardest days.

Thank you to my friend, Antonia, for being my daily source of support and insight as we navigate the world of rare disease together.

Thank you to my talented daughter, Rebecca, for helping me with my YouTube Channel and for being the best sister to Remy.

Thanks to all four of you for reading my book before I published it to offer critiques sandwiched by complements.

Thank you to my dad, Warren, for instilling my passion for spreadsheets and statistics.

Thank you to my son, Remy, for showing me what bravery looks like and for forcing me to become a better chef.

Thank you to Dr. Amy Myers, whose book *The Autoimmune Solution* led me on the path to my own healing.

Thank you to Dr. S, Dr. H and Dr. P for collectively saving my son's life.